SUPERCHARGED
SELF
HEALING

About the Author

RJ Spina has devoted his adult life to teaching people how to raise their frequency, improve the quality of their life, heal themselves, and experience the blissful state of truly being free.

He'd spent the better part of his life exploring profound metaphysical truths through his own higher consciousness exploration, but it was waking up from emergency life-saving surgery still permanently paralyzed from chest-down paralysis that awakened him to the highest truth he'd ever encountered: he could heal himself and walk again. It was something that he *instantaneously knew*. And he knew how he would do it.

> My body was destroyed, but I was free. It was as if my old operating system of awareness had been replaced with a greatly enhanced model with far greater receptivity, bandwidth, and processing ability. I knew immediately and precisely how I would heal myself. I was in a state of Grace and cosmic consciousness. I was truly free.

Within two months RJ was walking with the help of a physical therapist. On the one hundredth day after surgery, just as he had originally predicted on the very first day after emergency life-saving surgery, he was walking on his own. All the conditions he'd been diagnosed with—diabetes, pancreatitis, Hashimoto's disease, hypothyroidism, and a syndrome called autonomic dysreflexia—had been resolved. He uses the word *resolved* instead of *healed* because health requires maintenance, and when people think of themselves as "healed," they often return to the disharmonious habits that created the illness.

RJ has helped countless people. He has written dozens of articles about consciousness, the Greater Reality, meditation, the ability to project one's consciousness, and the nature of the Self. He teaches meditation, self-realization, self-healing, and how to become a healer to seekers around the world. His website is https://www.ascendthe frequencies.com, and the Ascend the Frequencies Instagram (https://www.instagram.com/ascendthefrequencies12/) has more than twenty thousand followers.

FIRST EDITION
Ninth Printing, 2024

Cover design by Shannon McKuhen
Interior art © Mary Ann Zapalac on pages 116, 117, 120, 121, and 123; all other art by the Llewellyn Art department

Llewellyn Publications is a registered trademark of Llewellyn Worldwide Ltd.

Library of Congress Cataloging-in-Publication Data
Name: Spina, RJ, author.
Title: Supercharged self-healing : a revolutionary guide to access high-frequency states of consciousness that rejuvenate and repair / by RJ Spina.
Description: First edition. | Woodbury, Minnesota : Llewellyn Worldwide, Ltd, [2021] | Summary: "This book presents a seven-step program sharing self-healing principles and techniques for working at higher frequencies in order to realize better health, vitality, inner peace, and freedom"— Provided by publisher.
Identifiers: LCCN 2021029204 (print) | LCCN 2021029205 (ebook) | ISBN 9780738768090 (paperback) | ISBN 9780738768250 (ebook)
Subjects: LCSH: Mental healing.
Classification: LCC RZ400 .S56 2021 (print) | LCC RZ400 (ebook) | DDC 615.8/528—dc23
LC record available at https://lccn.loc.gov/2021029204
LC ebook record available at https://lccn.loc.gov/2021029205

Llewellyn Worldwide Ltd. does not participate in, endorse, or have any authority or responsibility concerning private business transactions between our authors and the public.

All mail addressed to the author is forwarded but the publisher cannot, unless specifically instructed by the author, give out an address or phone number.

Any internet references contained in this work are current at publication time, but the publisher cannot guarantee that a specific location will continue to be maintained. Please refer to the publisher's website for links to authors' websites and other sources.

Llewellyn Publications
A Division of Llewellyn Worldwide Ltd.
2143 Wooddale Drive
Woodbury, MN 55125-2989
www.llewellyn.com

Printed in the United States of America

SUPERCHARGED
SELF
HEALING

A Revolutionary Guide to Access High-Frequency
States of Consciousness That Rejuvenate and Repair

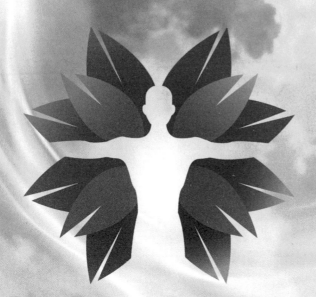

RJ SPINA

Llewellyn Publications · Woodbury, Minnesota

Disclaimer

Dedication

This book is dedicated to everyone, everywhere, who is suffering, and to those who compassionately care for all of those who cannot care for themselves. Also, to all the souls who have so courageously endeavored to have the human experience.

I dedicate it to the Masters who test their divine perfection, iron will, and cosmic consciousness in their efforts to free and lead humanity. And above all else, it is dedicated to the One Spirit that moves through all of existence.

May this book serve its highest purpose: the Victory of the Light.

Note: This book was written from what I experience directly through a state of higher consciousness, clarity, connectivity, and communion. These pages do not contain any beliefs or non-beliefs, but rather my direct personal experiences as well as the true stories of those who utilized the Ascend the Frequencies Healing Technique I developed to bring my permanently paralyzed and destroyed body back to life. I love you all more than you will ever know.

I am your holy brother,
RJ

Contents

Figures

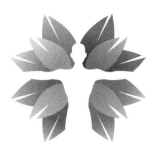

Foreword

By Adrian Bean, MSOTM, LAc

I first treated RJ at perhaps his lowest point. He was paralyzed from the chest down, and his surgeon told him to get used to it because he'd never seen a patient recover. It was four days after he'd undergone emergency spinal surgery to remove a sizable infection that had pressed against his cord, causing complete paralysis from the mid-back down. He had rampant diabetes and severe thyroid dysfunction as well. In addition to invading the spine, the lethal infection had completely overwhelmed his immune system, causing a severe autoimmune response. I am an acupuncturist and have treated over seventy-five thousand patients in my twenty-five years as a clinician. I also practice visceral manipulation and cranial osteopathy, a lineage emphasizing anatomically precise manual palpation skills. We work directly with nerves, organs, arteries, fascia and ligamentous tissues, bones, joints, etc. We also work directly with the brain and spinal cord. Once connected, we can then directly interact with the various tissues of the body, helping restore proper function. As I assessed RJ, his status was beyond grim: the crushed spine had caused the complete chest-down paralysis, the inflamed pancreas, the retracted heart, the enlarged and nodular thyroid. Multiple systems were overrun and essentially broken.

I was utterly astounded by another specific feature. I could directly feel that he was totally fine. His Soul was unscathed by the severe condition of his body. Early during the first session, as I worked with his brain and spinal cord to help restore flow through the damaged region, I had my hand on the crown of his head. After decades of practice and experience, I can differentiate various qualities of the brain and nerves. As I felt his head, expecting to feel his brain, I encountered a vast empty space. It was absolutely vacant and silent. Of the tens of thousands of patients I have treated during my long career as a health practitioner, I have never encountered this quality. The only way I can describe it is as authentic enlightenment.

RJ was fully cognizant of the adversity and razor clear that his Will would manifest his total healing. I have often encountered optimism in patients battling against steep odds, but this was completely different. He was simultaneously totally focused on walking and healing while being completely at peace with his severely compromised condition. He exuded full acceptance while all his energy was focused on healing. Within three weeks, he wiggled a toe; within three months, he was walking, exactly as he had predicted. His recovery was not at all linear: it was rapid, with multiple quantum leaps. Not only was the permanent chest-down paralysis healed, but his diabetes and thyroid dysfunction were also resolved. I have never seen this degree of transformation, let alone in such a short time. While I regularly witness dramatic improvements in my patients, if I hadn't witnessed this myself, I would consider it humanly impossible.

This illustrates part of his profound and almost unexplainable skill set: healing.

As I treated RJ over the following months, we became friends. Working on him was unique because he could directly feel and utilize my skill, intention, and perspective. Another rarity was that he was teaching me about energetics while I worked on him, rather than the other way around.

I discovered that we share some common ground. I teach patients meditation and ways to use their intention to promote healing. I work to free people from their limiting mindset and unleash their power so their body can heal. On a daily basis, I appeal to them not to squander their energy in thought and negativity, but to gather it and direct it into the cells and tissues. People need to get out of their own way. RJ has truly conquered this.

RJ is also masterful with energy. Many people like myself can move and gather qi. RJ is operating on an entirely different level. He has fully emptied himself. He doesn't think. He simply knows. Because of the nature of his Being, he has access to very high-frequency energy. This "Intelligent Energy," as he calls it, is unlike any qi I have encountered. We don't have this in common; here RJ stands alone. Over my lifetime, I have interacted with shamans, yogis, qi gong masters, mediums, and healers. RJ is unlike any being I have ever met, and his wisdom, perspective, and abilities extend far, far beyond anything I have ever experienced or thought possible.

I was given the gift of witnessing and participating in RJ's healing. As he met the massive challenges with grace, he was blessed with physical healing and expanded energetic power. I continue to benefit from the collaboration as I am elevated by it.

Adrian Bean, MSTOM, LAc; owner, Pacific Center of Health, San Diego, CA; award-winning acupuncturist and State of California Acupuncture Board member who co-creates and grades the California Acupuncture State Licensing Exam; certified in numerous modalities, including visceral manipulation, craniosacral therapy, and neural manipulation

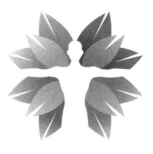

Introduction

Welcome, my friends. Chances are you're reading this book because you seek true liberation. Maybe you want to heal a physical issue, mental suffering, emotional trauma, or perhaps even a disease. I want you to understand that this journey is much bigger than even that. Fasten your seatbelt, because this is a giant leap forward in the evolution of individual and collective consciousness. You're about to learn the same steps that I took to heal my permanent chest-down paralysis as well as the myriad of diseases and catastrophic health issues I was diagnosed with.

Before we get into the spiritual physics of self-healing directed by the higher consciousness, I want to share with you something that is quite personal. When I was a child, I would normally and without any effort be able to see beyond the veil of our physical senses. I remember explaining to my mother that when I lay down to sleep at night, I would wake up in other realms outside of this world. At the very beginning of these experiences I would close my eyes, and in a moment I was pure spirit once again. My consciousness was outside of my body, and I would literally watch myself sleep. Sometimes I was floating above my body, and other times I was standing beside my bed. This quickly progressed, with my consciousness effortlessly roaming our house, neighborhood, or even local mountaintops.

I realized that, without any physical effort, my spirit could go anywhere. My lack of earthly attachment to being human and a focused intention were all that was required to catapult my consciousness into much higher realms of existence. I began to interact with advanced beings and their realities. My daily and nightly adventures afforded me a significantly deeper understanding of our mind/body/spirit and how they work in relation to the unseen world. It became totally normal for me to experience the seemingly unimaginable and to retain the depth of these magical wonders and their timeless wisdom.

When I told my mom about leaving my body and traveling in the unseen world, she had absolutely no idea what I was talking about. I really thought what I was doing was totally normal, and for me, it was. I was shocked to hear that the exact opposite was true for her and basically everybody else. Me doing this sort of thing certainly wasn't encouraged, to say the least. So I ceased talking about it for roughly twenty years. In fact, for the most part, I stopped actively doing it. It wasn't until I was twenty-four years old that I started to intellectually understand what I had been doing naturally and effortlessly as a child. Since then, I have spent the last twenty-five years of my life deconstructing, exploring, explaining, and teaching what I instinctively did as a child.

With that brief recapping of my history in mind, let's fast-forward to near present day. After being discharged from my two-month hospital rehabilitation stay as a result of an unexplained catastrophic septic shock that ravaged my body, and still paralyzed from the chest down, I was warned that my brittle rib cage was about to snap due to the physical exertion I was perpetually putting my body through in order to regain sensation and functionality from the chest down. I knew this physical exertion was an essential component in the journey to overcome my "permanent" chest-down paralysis. This was my response to that dire warning my health practitioner had given me: "I am willing to break everything in order to put myself back together."

I share this so everyone will understand the mindset of total victory. Authentic repair, true healing, and spiritual transcendence of great energetic disharmony and physical dysfunction are often beyond brutal. Your repair and healing will be the biggest challenge you have ever given yourself. It will be filled with overwhelming fear, constant physical turmoil, and emotional upheaval. There will be countless disheartening setbacks, sometimes painful rehabilitation injuries, and less than encouraging medical updates. Ultimately, the entire journey of healing is a crushingly lonely, individual endeavor.

But I am here to tell you that you are not alone.

The answer to your overcoming all of this disharmony and suffering begins with knowing that none of these phenomena are *you*. If you can perceive it, it cannot be you. You are what perceives. Woven within the very fabric of your perception is your depth of wisdom and love. That is the real you. That is what eternally exists prior and gives life to the voice inside your head, your body, and any disharmony it experiences.

No one is going to overcome your obstacles for you, because they cannot. See ill health for what it is: a challenge. Nothing more and nothing less. Accept it without hesitation so you can summon true grace and real power. I am going to show you how to remain supremely focused on your task. Never doubt that it won't be achieved. Do not leak your energy on any possibilities but your triumph. Never waver. What was once seemingly impossible will eventually be your manifested reality of victory if you refuse to give in.

Many people with chronic illnesses, addiction issues, and various physical, mental, or emotional traumas that weren't healed through other modalities have experienced a significant improvement in their well-being by practicing the Ascend the Frequencies Healing Technique (ATFHT). These people have experienced firsthand that healing comes in many forms even beyond the physical, and that authentic healing does not exist outside of themselves but rather within.

My personal self-healing journey is medically documented and captured on video because I knew nobody would believe this was possible. I am eternally devoted to helping others heal and liberate themselves using the same wisdom and techniques that I used. The seven-step Ascend the Frequencies Healing Technique captures exactly what I did to transcend the human ego/mind/identity (what I simplify to call the ego, ego mind, or egoic identity) and heal my entire body of energy. With the ATFHT, everyone and anyone who's sick, suffering, or seeking true ascension can now avail themselves of what has been, up until now, outside the collective consciousness.

All components of the ATFHT take the current understanding, application, and efficacy of neural rewiring and expound and enhance it by an order of magnitude. We are going to address how to access and cleanse our entire body of energy, and not just the more obvious lower sensory realms, by authentically activating our higher consciousness. This revolutionary understanding goes well beyond the mental reconfiguration of beliefs. You will learn how to powerfully redirect the same energy you use every day to think, emote, act, and behave for your healing, whether it's physical, emotional, mental, or spiritual.

My transcendence of permanent paralysis and severe ill health is your permission slip to do the impossible for your Self. You would not have this book in your hands if you were not ready. Let's begin.

How to Use This Book

Remember, true healing is not a mental exercise, emotional indulgence, or physical exertion. We often mentally comprehend what's wrong but can't change our state of being or ill health. Surrender is the key to unlocking your full potential. You must become one with the Self in order to powerfully command the divine process of healing as explained in this book. When we talk about surrender, I mean completely, not just mentally, emotionally, or physically. Never reach for a result, but rather endlessly flow with the creative process itself. Working with these steps will help.

The Steps of the Ascend the Frequencies Healing Technique

As you do the exercises in this book, dwell within the Self, your essence, not in thought, emotion, or physical tension, and watch what happens to your general state of being and health. We'll get more into how to go about doing this in chapter 2 and step 1. Being free, being the Self, will become your new habit. It makes for a far greater quality of life, the only true quality of life. I will guide you on your return to what is original to you: divinity, freedom, harmony, and perfection.

By utilizing the Ascend the Frequencies Healing Technique, the ego/mind/identity that is troubled by the body's ill health begins to lose sway over the Self's eternal freedom and perfection, and with it, so does its programs of ill health. The wisdom contained within this book is needed in order for you to drop many preconceived notions about healing.

Most of us are unwilling to change our habits (beliefs, thoughts, emotions, actions, and behaviors) in order to become well and liberated. Step 1, and your tangible understanding of it, is essential for your liberation and healing. It is crucial to tangibly see the egoic identity, and you will, in order to break its hold over your completeness and perfection. The efficacy of the protocols in step 1 are immediately palpable. True union with any remaining step, once step 1 has been mastered, will yield incredible results. Here is a summary of the full ATFHT program. This summary of the steps and their practices is repeated in even more detail in the book's conclusion, starting on page 173. This is a good page to bookmark for easy access as you move through the program.

Step 1: Access Your True Essence—Let go of your ego/mind/identity and access your true essence. These simple yet immensely powerful and transformative protocols dissolve the illusion of the ego/mind/identity, which is the root cause of all suffering and ill health. The core exercises help you connect with your true essence.

Step 2: Know Specifically What You Are Going to Achieve—Separate from your doubts and know specifically what you are going to achieve. You'll ask yourself the question "What specifically do I want to achieve?" and refine your answer multiple times through repeat questioning. The more fine-tuned and specific your answer, the more power you can harness to bring your specific desire into manifestation.

Rather than doubting, you can marry yourself to the vibration of victory already within you. This step will help you learn how to never waver in your conviction, so that the tangible recognition of your intention and desire must manifest. Once the desired achievement is written, the energetic contract is always in force, unless you willfully break it.

Step 3: Activate Your Healing Intention—Activate the state of healing with the intention you created in step 2. You will see (imagine), feel, perform, and verbalize your action. This step utilizes all fundamental human expression (mental, emotional, physical, and verbal) and activates the higher frequencies of intention/desire. This step can be thought of in this way: mental visualization + physical action + emotional stimulation + the spoken word = full activation of your healing intention.

Step 4: Command Creator Consciousness—You will learn how to access higher states of consciousness. This step provides the ultimate high-frequency meditation where you can access the hidden realms within the higher mind of Source. Higher consciousness is the chemist of our biology and the architect of our form. Accessing and commanding this high-frequency energy helps to repair and heal at the root and not just treat symptoms. Like an Etch A Sketch, access your higher consciousness and re-create yourself based upon what is original to you—the blueprint of perfection.

Step 5: Channel Intelligent Energy into the Body—You will learn how to access Intelligent Energy by channeling it into your body through the crown chakra. Follow the instructions in order to open your crown chakra and command or download Intelligent Energy into and through your entire body of energy. You can also have the Intelligent Energy pour out of your mini palm chakras and/or heart chakra and into any body part, organ, or system that needs repair. This Intelligent Energy has the innate ability to transmute and deprogram lower-frequency disharmony, which repairs and heals you.

Step 6: Turn Off the Program of Illness—Here you will learn how to turn off, unplug, and sever the connections to illness, like you would unplug and take down a neon sign. By accessing the higher frequencies (where the building blocks of our form and function exist), we learn to apply step 6 to literally turn off the program of illness we are running.

Symptoms are simply the tangible subset of various types of mis-programming we acquire and run called illness and disease. Like any mis-programming, these abnormalities were added and therefore can be turned off and deleted. Your mind/body complex (biological computer) runs best with the least amount of non-native programs running on its hard drive. No different from turning off a light and unplugging it from its power source, once done, the light is permanently off. The same is true when we turn off and delete the program of illness we are running. The illness no longer has an energy source to sustain itself.

Step 7: Use the Power of the Spoken Word—Here you will utilize the ancient power within the spoken word for repair, self-healing, and a greater quality of life. You can reharmonize your entire body of energy through commands, mantras, and affirmations. You'll learn how to let your Self's supremely high vibration regain total dominion over your incarnation by verbalizing your divinity, perfection, freedom, and victory.

Vibration, or sound, has been used for therapeutic purposes throughout antiquity, and true healers have continued to use it ever since. Our most powerful vibration is the internal dialogue we speak directly from the Self to our conscious mind and body of energy. Lower-frequency disharmony cannot exist within a supremely high-vibrational environment. As Buddha is believed to have said, "What we think, we become. What we imagine, we create. What we feel, we attract." Expression through speech can ensure your complete victory and liberation from disharmony.

Upon mastering and embodying the wisdom within step 1, complete dedication to any single step within the ATFHT can yield significant results in repair and healing and a far greater quality of life. Initially, do each of the steps in sequential order to familiarize yourself with all of the healing technique's components. At that point, you may be drawn to certain specific steps you wish to utilize frequently. All steps result in the tangible, direct experience of your true Self and the regaining of command over more and more of your energy. The mastery of multiple components within the ATFHT exponentially increases your power, transcendence, repair, healing, quality of life, and liberation.

How Long to Practice

We can look at the frequency and duration of performing any of the steps like we would approach a physical workout regimen or a meditation, yoga, or martial arts discipline. Forty-five minutes of complete union and dedication daily to any single step will produce great results. The beauty of the ATFHT is that you can do the steps for far more than forty-five minutes without ever getting exhausted. The more you let go as you give yourself over to the process itself, the more of your vitality (energy) returns, the healthier and more powerful you become in every way. Even three twenty-minute sessions dedicated daily to a single step would be a great start. Extending your consciously directed parasympathetic state for longer durations greatly increases self-healing efficacy. Let your enhanced quality of inner peace, expanded consciousness, and tangible freedom from disharmony be your criteria.

You Can Do This!

Many of us can get thrown off by self-care. That is because we are so used to being out of balance and aggressive with ourselves, even with our own healing. Any return of true inner balance feels odd. Powering through things ultimately leaves us drained of energy. When doubt that you can do this rears its head, simply ask yourself, "Who is it that doubts?" Your answer will be, "Me. I am the one who doubts." Then ask yourself, "Who am I?" You will get no answer. The mind will go blank. That's because the voice inside your head, the egoic identity, is not you. It's just a looped program of limitations. We are going to learn how to make that character disappear, and a superior quality of life will be revealed.

As you do the work properly, your vibration rises. That is exactly how healing and a greater quality of life works. Low-frequency disharmony cannot exist within a high-frequency environment. The Self, your essence, is a supremely high frequency. By attuning the brain, which the body must then follow, to the supreme vibration of the Self, healing occurs. Some of our new understandings will shine a much-needed light upon the idea of looking and straining for results. Exertion and forced effort keep us from accessing our innate balance and inner harmony.

It is essential to understand that it's the egoic identity alone who has the poor quality of life, whether the body is sick or not. The Self—what you really are—is formless, free, and unconditioned. My physical body was destroyed, permanently paralyzed from the chest down, wracked with incomprehensible pain, severe chronic illness, and life-threatening conditions, yet I was in a state of grace. I did not suffer. More accurately, I was in a state of cosmic consciousness, and my healing was a direct result of this.

Once the egoic identity has less of a stranglehold on the Self and its body of energy, the ailments that we are the awareness of do not impede our quality of life like before. We have space through the freedom of non-identification. That "work" space is needed in order to repair and heal. It is always about the quality of our inner life, because the outer life is not the Self. Not only do we learn how to repair and heal our body of energy—and healing comes in many forms—but we also learn how to free ourselves from the tyranny of the egoic identity. This is why the ATFHT is revolutionary.

All of us have a much nobler purpose than just the prolonging of our physical life. It is time to find this out for your Self. It's the only way to truly know anything. As the egoic identity disappears, the one who is troubled disappears as well.

As stated earlier, healing comes in many forms, and the physical is only one of them. Sometimes we sign up for instantaneous healing, fast healing, gradual healing, slow healing, or even no healing. That is because we must first address our higher-vibrational misperceptions, misunderstandings, and misidentifications. Nothing originates in the physical, and that is why there is nothing curative in this realm. It's not punishment; it's just how the game of self-realization is played. It's time to play it like a master!

I wrote this book so we can all begin to remember how to transcend suffering, the constraints of the human condition, and enjoy a greater quality of life. To be able to repair and heal ourselves, as well as each other, is eternally within each of us. It's really about the freedom of authentic self-realization in the form of a prescriptive book on how to repair, heal, and transcend disharmony and ill health. Liberation, freedom, and perfection are your destiny and birthright. Each one of you is the physical manifestation of that birthright.

Healing comes in many forms, and whatever form it begins with is of no consequence. What *is* important is that your liberation from suffering is manifested here and now. Trust in your Self so completely and utterly that fear and doubt no longer exist. You are more powerful than you can possibly imagine. We are all a spark of the infinite, a light that shines eternally, a life stream that continues infinitely. Your freedom from the self-imposed prison of your belief-based egoic identity and its disharmonious body of energy is how you heal and transcend. This transcendence, this freedom, is the Victory of the Light.

If you are scared or doubt yourself in any way, simply close your eyes, reach out, and take my hand. It's always there. I have pledged my eternal existence to the freeing of humanity. I shall remain here, for you, in freedom, love, and triumph for all eternity.

You have my unwavering devotion and attention, always.

I am your holy brother,

RJ

Part 1
The Fundamentals of the ATFHT

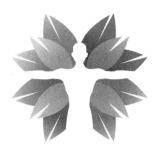

Chapter 1

Understanding the Invincible, Total You

My body is paralyzed, but what I am is not.

That was the realization that allowed me to transcend limitations and enter a state of consciousness where I knew how to heal myself.

In the spring of 2016, I was diagnosed with spinal subdural *Staphylococcus aureus* abscess, a lethal infection that compressed my spine and permanently paralyzed my body from the chest down. At the time, there were only sixty-five reported cases of this condition, and nobody who'd had it had regained full mobility and nearly all had died.

I was also diagnosed by the hospital's endocrinologist with type 1 diabetes, pancreatitis, Hashimoto's autoimmune disease, and hypothyroidism. I also experienced a condition called autonomic dysreflexia (AD), which is something that occurs most commonly with people who have a spinal cord injury above the sixth thoracic vertebra. My symptoms included a pounding headache, profuse sweating, and total nasal congestion that made breathing erratic and extremely difficult. Sudden and uncontrollable spikes in blood pressure, together with a rapid heartbeat and constricted blood vessels, increased my risk of having a stroke, cardiac arrest, loss of consciousness, and other life-threatening events. From the perspectives of the medical professionals, things looked bleak. I was told that if I survived, I would never walk again and would absolutely need several medications for the rest of my life. Good thing I didn't listen.

PREOPERATIVE DIAGNOSIS:
Thoracic spinal cord compression from epidural infection with (complete paraplegia.)

POSTOPERATIVE DIAGNOSIS:
Thoracic spinal cord compression from epidural infection with (complete paraplegia.)

PROCEDURE PERFORMED:
1. A T5 to T9 decompressive laminectomy with excision and removal of extradural dorsal epidural abscess.
2. Intraoperative use of fluoroscope.

Figure 1: Post-Surgical Notes

When my neurosurgeon told my partner at the time, Jennifer, the infectious disease doctor, and me about the chest-down paralysis being permanent, I was completely calm. Instead of feeling horrified at what the expert told me, I was free. I was experiencing what lies beyond samadhi (a term used to describe the transcendence of the cycle of birth and death). I was in a state of grace and total liberation from the human condition. I was free from any misperceptions, misunderstandings, or misidentifications. Instead of feeling like a prisoner in an immobile and diseased body, my consciousness took flight. I was completely detached from the prison of the finite mind and physical body. In this state of cosmic consciousness, I instantaneously knew how to heal myself, and the first thing I said to Jennifer was, "I will walk again. And even if I don't, I am at peace with everything." In that moment, even though she was worried and overcome with grief, she didn't doubt that I'd do what I vowed to do.

Today, I have conquered "permanent" paralysis and the myriad health issues have been resolved, but far more importantly I'm free. I'm free from the limitations that I'd previously created and accepted. To be more precise, I am free from what I call the ego/ mind/identity, which throughout this book I will call the *egoic identity*. That is the false, belief-based "I" that simultaneously identifies itself with the physical body. In a cosmic instant, I gained an entirely new understanding of Self, ill health, healing, and what we accept as so-called reality.

I understood that the Self, which is the screen of consciousness and whose fabric is our individual depth of love and wisdom, is what I eternally am. It's what we all are, love and wisdom, along with a complement or body of energy we are given. This energy we are given, like gas in a gas tank, is what we use to create things, like thoughts, emotions, physical actions, and experiences. The physical body is just a temporary vehicle for consciousness—the Self—to explore the physical universe with. This Self—or sentience—along with the complement of energy it is given, is what I call the Total Self. In other words, what we have always referred to as the soul is actually two very distinct parts: sentience, which is what we really are, and the complement of energy we are given to create with. When the Total Self is directly experienced, the door to higher consciousness and the Greater Reality, both of which exist within you but beyond our sensory perceptions and finite mind, is flung open.

Working with Your Higher Consciousness for Healing

You, too, will discover your own higher consciousness through this book, and this tangible realization will begin to liberate your body of energy from what it's holding onto, like ill health and sickness. Our consciousness is the gateway to the Greater Reality. This is what I did and why I know we are free. Everything we need to heal ourselves is at our command. So when I say that you possess everything you need to heal yourself, I am certain of this. The Self and its complement of energy is the cure for all that ails humanity. But don't believe me. Experience it firsthand, because that's the only way we ever really know anything.

Directly experiencing the Self, your own higher consciousness, and the Greater Reality will require you to suspend judgment and disconnect from the limitations that the finite mind creates by thinking. Your consciousness is an individualized or biological blueprint of the multiverse, and we make a holographic impression upon it with every single moment of our existence. Like a box inside a smaller box, all of our individualized consciousness is nested within the collective consciousness, which is within the consciousness of the Creator.

I sometimes refer to it as Creator/Source instead of God, because the word God has become politicized (what hasn't?) and is associated with so many inaccurate meanings and intentions. Source, as I directly know it, created our Higher Selves, which created our Souls, which explore the physical universe by having the human experience. This same Creator, Source, or God always provides everything we need. Lack is but a concept born of limited understanding. Contrary to popular belief, Source/God/Creator does not judge us—we do that to ourselves and each other. Source unconditionally loves us, always. It learns about itself through its creations just as our Higher Self learns about itself through us, and we learn indirectly about the Self through our creation: the belief-based egoic identity and the temporary physical body. This is not a thought or belief but something to experience directly.

Speaking of thinking, we don't need to think in order to do the things we do on a daily basis. We see a chair and we remember how to sit. We see a drinking glass and recall how to drink from it. Ninety-nine percent of our daily existence falls into this category: memory. Thinking is actually a bad habit that keeps you perpetually locked in the past because *thinking is the movement of the past*. It's revisiting memories, experiences, and what has been learned. The so-called future is always based upon the past, and therefore what we call the future is nothing more than a limiting mental concept.

Thinking is faltering because it's a by-product of experiencing a low-frequency environment. When we experience the higher frequencies and dimensions (and I will show you how to do that) utilizing our higher consciousness, we know. When we experience the lower frequencies of the physical universe, we lose direct access to the Self, internal knowingness, so instead we think.

When we raise our personal frequency, we raise our level of awareness and understanding about the Total Self and our surroundings. Raising our frequency is like being given a ladder to peek over at a maze. As soon as we can peek over the walls, we don't need to figure the way out because we see the way out. Like a bolt of lightning, in that moment of recognition, we know. This provides a profoundly deeper and more holistic perspective. This action is the direct engagement of our sentience (the Self). But in the lower frequencies, we're still wandering around in our maze, trying to think our way out of it. It's thinking itself that prevents us from acquiring the ladder, and it's thinking that limits us to being merely human. Thinking is not knowing, and its progenitor is always beliefs.

While thinking misuses energy to revisit the past in order to project a future of limitations, imagining and creating uses our complement of energy to make something new. When we're operating within a defined parameter, our creativity is limited to those parameters. Applying what we've learned is a severely limited form of creativity, if it is one at all. If a hammer is the only tool we know how to use, we see everything as a nail.

In order to evolve consciousness with the greatest efficacy, we must experience freedom from what we think we know, which means leaving the past and its future. Now, not through a past or a future, is how we access the timeless depth of the immortal Self through its eternal wisdom and limitless imagination. This simultaneously gives us access to the Greater Reality as well. This is how the ATFHT was born, and this is how you will liberate, repair, heal, and greatly improve the quality of your life.

The instant you stop thinking, you'll disconnect from the limiting beliefs you have about yourself and the world. In that inner spaciousness is where the freedom to repair and heal yourself exists. I will show you how to disconnect the Self from its misidentification with the physical body and your belief-based egoic identity. This is how all true liberation and healing occurs. Only in freedom from the past or future does one experience the majesty of life directly. But that's just the beginning of our journey. While learning to repair and heal yourself, you will unfurl your consciousness and rediscover higher intuitive functions. The "you" that you thought you were will disappear, and what you eternally are will be experientially known. The statement "All healing takes place within" is an ancient truth, not a New Age adage. It's the Self that commands tangible transformation, and subsequently your body of energy experiences repair and healing.

Authentic healing never originates, nor does it take place, in just the lower frequencies of physical reality. This is why what passes as medicine today is not curative. It's like constantly drying your flooded basement while the leak is upstairs. When you stop blocking your own inherent divine intelligence, you simultaneously experience better health and greater joy, fulfillment, and inner peace.

You're Not Who You Think You Are

Our vulnerability to illness is due to our lack of direct, tangible Self-awareness and having full command of our body of energy. This includes the belief that we are the physical body and the belief-based egoic identity. We are easily fooled by this illusion because we constantly rely on the human vehicle, its five senses, and its belief-based thinking. Eventually we lose the immortal Self due to misidentification with the temporary human experience. Our misidentifications have a cumulative effect. Every belief, thought, emotion, and experience that we identify with further perpetuates a lack of self-awareness, and this creates greater disharmony within ourselves and with each other.

This occurs because we do not know how to break free from this temporary limiting condition. Most people believe they're a physical body and identify with its physical sensations, emotions, thoughts, and experiences. But we are none of those things. We give birth to these things as a creator being, but we are not these things. We are the awareness of all that is perceivable and the eventual understanding and mastery of the process of creation itself.

What I saw and experienced when I was permanently paralyzed is that the human experience is but a temporary creation for sentience, the Self, to evolve itself, and that a human's perceivable reality is less than 0.003 percent of the Greater Reality. To better navigate our infinitely larger playing field—our higher consciousness and the Greater Reality—the comprehension of the following terms is vital, as they pave the way for a new paradigm.

energy: The pure life force itself, or what has been referred to as the Holy Ghost, or qi. It simply is, it flows, and it represents the infinite potential of limitless possibility.

sentience/the Self: What we *really are*; timeless wisdom and unconditional love. A fractal of God/Creator/Source.

Soul/the Total Self: Sentience + a body of energy to create with = the Total Self. Our sentience manipulates its complement of energy in order to animate the body and create thought, emotion, action, behavior, etc. Humanity has previously lumped these two separate elements, sentience and energy, into one thing and referred to them as the Soul.

the Higher Self/Totality: This is the much larger being that we, our Soul/Total Self, is but a drop of. Our Higher Self is literally everything we have been, are, and will be. It is truly our Totality. This incomprehensibly massive body of sentience and energy exists well outside of space and time. As an analogy for incarnating, you can imagine an octopus (Higher Self/Totality) dipping one of its tentacles (Total Self/Soul) deeper into the water to experience what that specific level of water is like.

physical body/genetic entity: This is the human vehicle and our genetic entity. It's the perceiver and experiencer of the physical universe. The physical body protects the sentience, or Self, and affords it the temporary experience of physical reality. Nobody takes their physical body with them when their incarnation is over, because we are not the physical body nor do we need it except for incarnation. It is only needed to explore the lower frequencies of the physical universe. Think of it like the diving bell a deep-sea diver must adorn prior to diving into the deep water for the work needing to be done.

    I use the term "physical body" throughout because it helps to separate misidentification with "the body" as being who we are. The physical body is like the car we drive. The car is the vehicle; it isn't who we are but rather something we temporarily get inside of that gets us from point A to point B. Similarly, every car suffers wear and tear from its multiple drivers and total mileage. It works the same way, except on a significantly deeper way (think genetic/hereditary traits we inherit) that I will explain in detail later.

ego/ego mind/egoic identity/EMI (ego/mind/identity): The ego/mind/identity (EMI) is the belief-based human character that the Self creates through its cumulative misperceptions, misunderstandings, and misidentifications. It is the "who" we think we are and has been referred to as the ego, the ego mind, the egoic identity, the false self, the shadow self, and the shadow identity. More accurately, the belief-based egoic identity is a limitation program that runs by thinking. Sentience, what we really are, knows and loves. The egoic identity, the false character we create, only thinks and feels in context to its beliefs and attachments. All suffering is the domain of the egoic identity. All completeness, happiness, peace, and power resides outside of the assumptions, ruminations, and projections that the egoic identity creates.

❄ ❄ ❄

Essentially, our life on Earth is a temporary experience that was set into motion when our Higher Self, with its built-in directive for its own self-evolution, projected a piece of itself, the Total Self/Soul, almost like a drone, into the lower frequencies of the physical universe, thus enrolling us into what is known as the evolutionary cycle.

Our individualized evolution as a projection from our Higher Self, or our Totality, mandates our continual rebirth until the requisite sentience (love and wisdom) is accrued in order to evolve past the need to incarnate, but first we must ascend the frequencies. Each time we incarnate, the Total Self/Soul temporarily merges with a physical body, and in this low-frequency environment, consciously cut off from our Higher Self and its Creator, it begins to misidentify with the physical body and its limited sensory-realm perceptions. These woefully incomplete perceptions are the tiny data stream that creates the finite mind, which forms beliefs, thoughts, opinions, judgments, and so-called knowledge.

Every time the Self misidentifies with a belief, thought, emotion, action, or experience, it becomes part of our egoic identity. We hold this limitation, this false sense of self, in place like an energetic prison for our consciousness and body of energy, and we perceive every experience we have while incarnate through this lens of limitation—more accurately, *as* this limitation. This false limited-self, your belief-based egoic identity, is a self-imposed delusional state born of your misperceptions, misunderstandings, and misidentifications. These are all limitations and not what you are at all. You are not the character you have created. The painter is not the painting. You, sentience, are complete, divine, immortal, and Free. You, as an immortal creator being, have simply created your own limitations.

You Don't *Have* Sentience, You *Are* Sentience

When we decide to reincarnate, we do so within an evolutionary cycle while nested within the evolving collective consciousness. The cumulative experiences of one's Higher Self/Totality are not accessible through the finite mind, because it can't perceive anything frequentially beyond the limited data stream provided by the five physical senses, which are attuned to a very limited bandwidth within the lowest frequencies. Our physical eyes perceive light that exists only within the range of 430–770 hertz. Similarly, our ears perceive the vibration of light that exists only within the 20 hertz–20 kilohertz range. These are mere fractions of the entire light spectrum. In the truest sense, we see, hear, and therefore understand nearly nothing. Like a drop of water in the ocean, the Total Self is but a drop of our Totality in every way.

In order to experience the unlimited and divine, one must be in an unlimited and divine state.

As we said, our Higher Self/Totality resides in a significantly higher frequential environment, or "space" within the Greater Reality, than we experience here on Earth. A frequency is an assignation of energy. It is the rate at which energy vibrates within a specific environment, while a dimension is a larger framework that houses frequencies. We don't exist dimensionally but rather frequentially. Our Higher Self has no direct experience of the lower frequencies and therefore has no experience of what it's like to be cut off from Source/God/Creator, the Greater Reality, to feel separate, alone, confused, angry, lustful, jealous, cold, vengeful, indecisive, or prideful. It knows nothing of the physical sensations of touch, taste, smell, low-frequency emotions, physical sex, or even thoughts, vanity, greed, fear, or anger. Our Higher Self resides well outside of the physical universe, beyond space and time. In order for it to learn what this slow, heavy, dense environment feels like, it must project a piece of itself—you—into this frequency, or "frequential environment." While this occurs, our Higher Self puts itself into stasis so that its drone or creation—you, the Total Self—can learn and work on its behalf. For you to keep moving up the frequencies, you must evolve and master yourself—not the beliefs of the egoic identity— within every possible environment. This includes the lower frequencies of the physical universe where our version of Earth resides.

All higher intuitive functions reside within the higher consciousness aspect of our sentience, not in low-frequency belief-based intellectual meanderings or emotions. The life force we use to accomplish everything we do, including thinking, emoting, and doing, is the same energetic power that you'll use to liberate, repair, and heal yourself.

You—Sentience—Are Not the Physical Form

Your DNA holographically contains your ancestors past blended with yours. How you damage, heal, or enhance your genetics is determined by your vibration, more specifically, by every belief, thought, emotion, action, and behavior you choose moving forward. By transcending the lower consciousness belief-based programming and consciously accessing your divine will and therefore your true energetic power, which you will learn how to do later, you create the opportunity for profound healing on multiple levels, which permanently repairs and unlocks more of your untapped DNA. This is the gift and the responsibility we have as immortal creator beings. Presently, though, we have tasked ourselves with a physical body that quickly becomes ill, suffers from countless diseases and disorders, experiences an increasing lack of functionality, grows old, and easily dies. Why is that?

The "fall of humankind" describes humanity's drop in frequency, which happened because of our misidentification and preoccupation with the finite mind and physical body. Originally, we were directly and consciously connected to the Source of all (renewing) life within ourselves. The complement of energy we were given in order to think, emote, act, and create was not misused by trying to conquer, dominate, and control nature. The physical body, or genetic identity, remained harmonious and lived for ages because we maintained our inner perfection and connection to Source/God/Creator.

The disharmonious tangible body is the physical manifestation of our disassociation from the Self and its Source. It is also the tangible experience of the choices we have made that distance us from wisdom and love. Our direct connection to our Higher Self was once so robust that an energetic force field formed around us, surrounding and protecting us. This force field used to extend several feet beyond the physical body. Today, due to our drop in frequency, it has contracted to an invisible, tight tube. This tube has been referred to in Eastern writings as the "hara line." In some cases, just like a hospital quarantines the highly contagious in order to protect themselves and others from contamination, the disconnection we experience from our Higher Self can be nearly complete in order for it to protect itself from infection caused by the disharmonious energies of the egoic identity.

Each physical body is a combination of the DNA and cellular memories of the sperm and egg that co-create it. Additionally, the physical body is imbued with the misperceptions, misunderstandings, and misidentifications that we carry within our own body of energy—from all our incarnations. In this sense, the physical body is a collection of past impressions, memories, choices, and experiences. This collection is embedded in patterns of structured higher consciousness called "energetic templates." These templates are the true building blocks of form and exist outside of the lower frequencies of our physical perception. Our Higher Self uses a step-down frequential process, like a Slinky going down a staircase, to create the energetic templates that eventually get translated into RNA, DNA, proteins, and cellular structure of the physical body. Think of this as formless higher, supremely intelligent, diffused energy consciously expressing itself as form within the physical universe.

Our physical body, much like DNA, is a biological computer that contains the history, or programming, of every soul that ever incarnated into that specific genetic line. This includes the current soul residing within that specific physical body—you. Every belief, thought, emotion, action, behavioral pattern, and social programming is embedded within the DNA. We know and see this prior to our incarnation. We are never at the mercy of genetics. Victimhood does not exist. What is paramount to understand is that powerfully directed sentience, utilizing its full complement of energy, can override previous disharmonious programming and literally realign our energetic templates, which rewrites our genetic code.

We constantly alter our DNA through our *attention*. Where attention goes, energy flows. Every thought, emotion, action, and behavior literally rewrites our past, present, and future. Every single stimulus, even those that are imperceptible to our physical senses, affects our DNA. But it's sentience and every single choice it makes that has the most effect on our DNA. We could say that we're all here to understand and heal what we have set into motion while simultaneously fulfilling our personal destiny.

By using our higher mind, we can see the details within the structure of human form. It's obvious that the past and present are all contained within our energetic templates and eventually expressed as genetic code. As we raise our personal and collective frequency, we will gain conscious access to what exists outside of space and time. As we do this, we unlock more and more of our individual and collective potential.

For decades, the myth that DNA is fixed has prevailed, but new research is showing that practices like meditation and yoga can reverse DNA reactions that are triggered by stress.[1] (*Stress* is another word for *reacting*.) This is possible because what people think of as a physical body is simply a body of energy vibrating at a specific band of frequencies, and therefore it can be greatly altered and manipulated through the focused power of our higher mind.

Remember, sentience—what you really are—needs to be housed in a physical vehicle attuned to its local environment in order to experience and endure this heavy, dense frequency, just as a deep-sea diver needs a diving bell to survive and function while immersed in the depths of the sea. Our "diving bell" is our physical body, and our oxygen tank is our complement of energy. Unfortunately, with nearly zero conscious connection to our Higher Self, we no longer

....

1. Coventry University, "Meditation and Yoga Can 'Reverse' DNA Reactions Which Cause Stress, New Study Suggests," Science Daily, June 15, 2017, https://www.sciencedaily.com/releases/2017/06/170615213301.htm.

have our normal complement of wisdom, power, higher intuitive functions, mobility, or holistic awareness at our disposal. Therefore, sentience is forced to rely on the physical body's five outwardly focused and extremely limited senses, which were designed for physical survival and were never meant to be used to create a wholly discordant egoic identity.

Our five senses are not focused inward because we couldn't keep our body safe and intact very long if we ignored the dangers we face in the physical world. This is obvious and understood, but when we desire self-awareness, we must look within. And when we do, we discover something life-changing: we're not victims of our genetics. You can discover this for yourself, and when more of the scientific community understands this truth, our current paradigms of health and disease will be turned upside down and inside out. You, by reading this book, are way ahead of the curve.

My direct experience and understanding is that sentience chooses what it wants to experience and work with, which includes the specific physical body it incarnates into. Not only do we choose the body, but we also choose what frequency (what we currently misunderstand as dimensions), timeline, and which team we are going to play for. We are that powerful a creator being and we are that free. Therefore, we're never victims of anything except our own ignorance and arrogance, but certainly not genetics. The point is to become aware of our choices and to fully understand our motivation behind them. It is our choices that control and determine evolution or stagnation. Far more importantly, it's our choices that dictate the evolution or regression of the Self and our Higher Self.

Victimhood Is a Concept That Exists Only in the Unawakened Mind

Remember that DNA is the result of a frequential Slinky-like step-down translation from our energetic templates, which exist outside of our physical sensory perceptions and therefore our intellect. We can think of the energetic templates as structured higher thought patterns within the higher frequencies of pure creativity. I explain these templates in more detail later in the book, but for now what's important is that they are the true building blocks of form. That means, when accessing our higher consciousness, we can direct and dictate our self-repair and healing regardless of the hereditary lineage contained within the physical body we incarnated into. This is part of what I did to heal myself and help others, and what you are about to learn to do too. But first, we have some deconstruction work to do. Identifying the illusions awakens us to the truth.

The "I" That Isn't You

From the moment we're reborn into the lower frequencies of the physical universe, we begin to assemble a false identity. This is due to the loss of access to our own higher consciousness and normal high-frequency environment. Our near-total lack of tangible self-awareness while temporarily merged within a human vehicle, immersed and attuned to a low frequency with nonstop behavioral and societal programming, is beyond catastrophic to our consciousness. It causes total amnesia. This is how and why our egoic identity is formed. In fact, we are greatly encouraged to do just that—to create an egoic identity or risk not "fitting in." The absolute truth is there is no need to fit in, as you did not come here to stay. This separate belief-based "I" we are speaking about is the accumulation of your misperceptions, misunderstandings, and misidentifications. All that we perceive, including the physical body, that we have misidentified our Self with becomes part of our ego/mind/identity limitation program. It is always limiting, because whatever we choose to identify with is always a mere fraction of the completeness of the Self.

The belief-based egoic identity is born of the physical body's limited perceptions, which provide the data stream for the construction of our logic-and-linear-bound intellect. The Self misidentifies itself as the physical body and its highly mediocre capabilities. It believes in the limiting delusions it creates or were given. Since the physical body outwardly perceives only mere fragments of the Greater

Reality, we experience this fragmentation within ourselves. We then relate to the outside world through fragmentation—a separate "I." Perception becomes reality, so it follows that limited perception creates limited reality and therefore a limited sense of Self. This is precisely what the belief-based egoic identity is: a self-created limitation program that runs by thinking. We believe so deeply in the authenticity of our egoic identity program of limitations that it destroys all tangible recognition of the divine and complete Self within us all.

Remember, if you can perceive it, it cannot be you. You are perception itself.

Our egoic identity is created through the acceptance, misidentification, mimicry, and subsequent repetition of external stimuli: what we have believed in, what Mommy and Daddy said to us, what we were exposed to in school, what we have read and watched, thought and felt, experienced and remembered. None of these things touches what you really are…sentience.

Right now there are roughly 7.8 billion people in the world, and everyone thinks what they do is right. You can think of the belief-based egoic identity as a collection of filters that make it impossible to see or appreciate the divine within yourself, anyone, or anything. These filters make it impossible to see and experience anything for what it "is." If we do not understand the Self, how can we truly understand anything? Continually remind yourself (and soon I will share exercises that tangibly prove this) that the egoic identity is a self-imposed prison, a limitation program that runs by thinking. For now, as a test to prove just how controlled the Self is by the belief-based egoic identity, see how long you can go without it running its program of limitations. In other words, see how long you can go without thinking right now. Go ahead and stop reading and see how long you can go without thinking. A lack of self-control makes self-discipline impossible. This keeps self-healing and a superior quality of life firmly out of our tangible experience. You must transcend the bubble of your belief-based, physical perception of yourself, and we are going to learn how to do just that.

Your Higher Mind's Imagination

Instead of working with your egoic beliefs, you'll learn to work with your higher mind's imagination for healing. We often think of our false identity as "fixed." How many times have you said or heard someone say, "That's just who I am"? But it's not who we are at all. Don't we change our mind about things? Haven't we changed how we feel about something or someone? Haven't we changed our opinions, beliefs, habits, friends, professions, life partners, and where we live? Is there anything about our identity that is actually fixed? One can change a thousand times in a day and still be wearing the same clothes.

Scientists today have even discovered that what we experience as solid is actually 99.9999999 percent empty space.[2] Do you really think anything going on with your seemingly physical body is actually permanent? Every thought, feeling, and experience we ever have simply comes and goes like a breeze blowing through the room. It's all transient. All of it. Including illness.

But what is the one constant? The awareness of it—sentience— the Self. You. Just like a time-lapse camera unflinchingly watching, you are the awareness of the physical body, what it perceives, experiences, and processes. You are the eternal and immortal creative observer of the perpetual flow of change. You are not the physical body and what it experiences, nor are you the thoughts, feelings, or analysis of the constant stream of phenomena. You only "think" you are because your belief-based egoic identity runs a limitation program called thinking that includes identifying with the physical body itself. This misunderstanding makes you believe that you are your "body" and your false identity. It's only your belief in the authenticity of your created identity that makes it "real."

We know the egoic identity is an illusion born of habit because when we stop giving it attention, through authentic meditation, the

....

2. Ali Sundermier, "99.9999999% of Your Body Is Empty Space," Business Insider, September 23, 2016, https://www.businessinsider.com/physics-atoms-empty-space-2016-9.

false "I" disappears. The Self is meditation. That's when we experience true freedom and tangible peace. We also get all our energy back because that's the energy the egoic identity currently uses to attach itself to beliefs/thoughts/emotions/body/experiences. Once we have our complement of energy back, that is when we tangibly experience our completeness, divinity, joy, wisdom, and love. Now we are truly powerful once again.

Sentience—what you really are—does not suffer. Ever. Even if the body/mind is in a state of total disrepair. Only through misidentification does suffering occur. We only ever suffer our own lack of self-awareness. The only death we ever experience is the disconnection from the immortal Self within.

The belief-based egoic identity is designed to approach everything as a problem that needs a solution, because it is founded on limitations and incompleteness. If we approach a so-called terminal illness or permanent paralysis as a problem, we won't heal, because there is no solution for these "problems." So instead of misidentifying the immortal Self with the problem, I will show you how to simply work with "what is": your higher mind's unlimited imagination to potentially recreate what is already within—absolute harmonic perfection.

Physical Reality Is Temporary Tangible Form

Physical reality is temporary tangible form in order to understand the formless creator within. If life is a play, then our belief-based egoic identity is the character *playing us*. We can also use the analogy of a video game. Our Higher Self creates an avatar, which is the soul, in order to experience each level (frequency/reality) of the game on Earth and elsewhere. Every level in which we master ourselves enhances our avatar, and we move up to the next level. Similarly, the more our sentience deepens, the more access it has to higher functionality. As sentience deepens and accrues, the more energy we are given and can command. This leads to a more advanced Self and a similarly more advanced physical vehicle. This is ascension. More accurately, it is ascending the frequencies of the multiverse.

When the avatar clears all the levels and has mastered the Self within every environment, there is no need to experience this game again for evolutionary purposes. We have cleared all the boards, so to speak. Once self-mastery is realized, we move on to a completely different game and eventually master the Self in that new one as well. It never ends, but what does end is the need to incarnate into the lower frequencies. Instead, your Higher Self continues its never-ending journey to "know its limitless nature" by projecting the same or different pieces of itself (you) into even higher frequential realms of existence, where the directive of Self-mastery continues endlessly within those environments.

Where the linear, rational, and extremely limited human mind breaks down is in the idea that all of this—everything—is happening concurrently, simultaneously, and in parallel. There is only one moment of creation experienced from an infinite amount of perspectives. While incarnate in the lower frequencies, we simply do not have the proper vantage point, receptivity, and bandwidth (just like a radio can only tune in to one station at a time) to experience the vastness of simultaneous existence in a more holistic manner. Just as often, we don't have the requisite sentience to truly understand the concurrent/parallel/simultaneous totality of existence, but that doesn't mean it's not occurring and real.

Rather than investing your energy in something the finite mind can never experience nor comprehend, like the totality of all existence, instead use your intention to stop misidentifying with your disharmonious belief-based program of limitations. A far greater quality of life awaits you. We must detach or dissociate from our misidentifications in order to bring ourselves back to our naturally harmonious and joyous state. The health, freedom, and completeness that we all intrinsically possess can never be experienced by misidentifying the Self with our limiting egoic identity and temporary physical body.

Misidentifications are always limited and therefore always dishar-monious. Remember, the poet is not the poem. We experience these divine qualities within only upon freeing our Self from the tyranny of the low-frequency belief-based egoic identity and its misidentification with the physical body.

Misperceptions, misunderstandings, and misidentification are the source of all suffering, and everything other than unsullied awareness (sentience) is not you. You must let go of everything. The more you tangibly understand this, the more of your energetic power you will regain. This energy is needed to repair and heal yourself.

In chapter 2 you'll learn how to begin the process of "undoing" and disassociating with the physical body and the egoic identity.

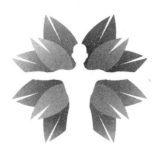

Chapter 2

Let Go of Belief and Access the Magic of Your Imagination

Creation, like the blossoming of a lotus flower, is silent. Destruction, like the tearing down of a tree, is loud. Do not fear the deconstruction of your disharmonious, belief-based egoic identity and its misprogrammed body of energy, no matter how loud and unsettling the process. It must go in order to command the experience of harmony and perfection already within you.

Being ill isn't a form of punishment, and it's certainly not God's will. It's simply a self-mastery challenge over our body of misprogrammed energy. Blame does not exist either, except within the feckless flailing of duality. There is simply feedback based upon choices. Ultimately, there is only what works and what doesn't work in terms of what we are trying to achieve. Your mission is to awaken from the spell of this low-frequency environment, and through tangible self-awareness vanquish the egoic identity, take full command of your body of energy, and thus return to what is the Original You: health, vitality, power, and a tangible connection to the immortal and divine Self.

The physical body has a limited form of consciousness all its own, but it must surrender to the far greater Sentience that is the

Self. You, sentience, command the body. If we do not utilize our innate wisdom and love, then we are operating with only fragmentary data from our low-frequency physical senses. This keeps us in the limited realm of body consciousness, which is identification with the physical body and its poor sensory perceptions. In turn we become victims to genetics and the limitations of so-called knowledge. Authentic self-healing cannot take place within any delusional state. Neither can true peace, joy, and happiness.

One of the fundamentals of self-repair and healing is recognizing that the knowledge and beliefs that are commonly accepted about health and healing are simply not true. In these higher consciousness realms, energy immediately responds to the pure force of imaginative intention. It does here in the physical universe as well, just much more slowly. That way, we can see ourselves in the act of creation. This is all part of perfecting our abilities as master creators.

To help with separation from the body, it's the physical body, not our Sentience, or what we really are, that responds to muscle testing. Same with eating in accordance with our blood type. These responses of the body have nothing to do with Sentience. We, sentience, are the awareness of the body's reaction to muscle testing and the effect of our dietary habits.

Despite this truth, most people believe they are the physical body, outer personality, and everything they've temporarily accumulated. I am the sum of all of these things, and the more I lay claim to both the tangible (money and stuff) and the intangible (knowledge and experiences), the bigger, more important, more successful, and worthy my egoic identity becomes. In this belief system, "the more I have, the more I am."

There are also people who believe that by shunning material possessions and earthly knowledge, they've destroyed their ego. But shunning is just the flip side of acquiring. They are two sides of the same coin. Duality is the domain of lower frequencies and births the belief-based egoic identity. Freeing Sentience—our timeless, immortal awareness—from the tyranny of our linear, logical mind and limiting body consciousness is the only real revolution that ever takes place. All of our power is in getting our energy back from the egoic identity.

The physical body can be repaired and healed once we no longer identify with it. Think of it this way: we cannot transcend what we refuse to let go of. Our new and more holistic understanding of the Sentience (the Self), its complement of energy, and the temporary human experience is a leap forward in the evolution of sentience and humanity's subsequent healing. Only in the deconstruction of the belief-based egoic identity does true healing and a superior quality of life take place.

Override the Ego/Mind/Identity Limitation Program

Healing requires overriding energetic misprogramming, so the first step in the Ascend the Frequencies Healing Technique (ATFHT) is the accessing of our true nature. This will cease the impetus driving your disharmony. You must apply the brakes first in order to release everything that has accumulated through misperceptions, misunderstandings, and misidentifications. This way, you can increase your functionality by rewiring your entire misprogrammed energy field simply by returning to what is original to you. That vibration, the Self, is what you must use to heal your body of energy. The Self is an infinitely higher vibration than the low-frequency egoic identity and physical body, so it naturally harmonizes them and everything else in this much lower frequential plane of existence.

By consciously living as the Self, our entire body of energy naturally heals. But what's far more important with regard to your journey of Self-mastery is that living directly as the Self is the most expedient way to evolve. By refusing to misidentify with the egoic identity and physical body, I overrode their limitations of misprogramming, which included paralysis and severe chronic illness, and powerfully commanded my healing precisely as I had predicted.

It is worth repeating: the belief-based egoic identity is a limitation program that runs by thinking. It is constructed from fragments of the whole and is therefore always in need of something to complete itself. This perpetual wanting and ever-present incompleteness—the egoic identity is disharmony itself—can only produce disharmonious thought patterns, which are the source of health problems. All disharmony, when taken back to its energetic inception and conception, comes from disharmonious thought patterns. We cannot expect the source of our ill health—belief-based thinking—to fix our ill health.

To better understand the egoic identity, imagine a racetrack with disharmonious thoughts racing around the track like cars. The more cars there are and the faster they travel, the more disharmony, chaos, and collisions occur, which results in increased sickness, disease, and malfunctions. And since the belief-based egoic identity is an endless loop of misperceptions, misunderstandings, and misidentification, there is no end to this race and we can never win. But we *can* disassociate with the cars and rise above the racetrack. From that frequential perspective, we can heal the damage that we've done below.

What we *can't* do is heal ourselves with our egoic identity, because it's the source and creator of problems. The egoic identity is a master at imbuing disharmony. We bathe thoughts in emotion through identification with thoughts. This act of bathing thoughts with energy through identification with them creates feelings. These feelings about ourselves and others are what cause our suffering. The egoic identity has nothing to do with *what* we truly are. It's just a creation, a character in a play. Your memorized dialogue is the collection of beliefs you have identified with, and beliefs are the context for every thought. Disharmonious thought patterns lead to disharmonious feelings, actions, experiences, and behaviors. But buried beneath the temporary construct of the egoic identity limitation program is wholeness and completeness, freedom itself, unending joy, timeless wisdom, and unconditional love with an indomitable power at its disposal. That's *what* you are, not a tiny *who*.

By misidentifying with our limited ego identity, we forfeit unlimited imagination—our true magick—in favor of a transient, disempowering reality. We literally give our life force, our energetic power, to the egoic identity. That's how we become slaves to the concepts, beliefs, memories, and information that we've misidentified with, including the physical body. Everything we place our attention on or allow into our environment greatly affects our energy field and our health. Every sound, image, and vibration. Everything. Even stimuli that the physical body and finite mind can't consciously perceive have a profound effect on us. Have you ever suddenly become aware of a sound and realized it's been going on for a while? Though you just became aware of it, you were still affected by it. These energies leave impressions within our body of energy and have a massive impact upon us even though consciously we are completely unaware of them.

This understanding has far-reaching implications. We must summon our will to detach from the trancelike egoic identity that is built upon the delusion of beliefs. It is the only way we can tangibly see these energetic constructs for what they really are: the enslavement of our immortal consciousness that is yearning and designed for the freedom of unlimited imagination within the higher mind of God/Source/Creator.

We're Designed with the Capacity to Heal Ourselves

Trying to conquer nature through thought, which is what we call scientific progress, has been a perpetual outward expenditure of our energy, which only leads to the medicalization of health. Our inner nature is harmony and balance and is reawakened prior to thought itself.

The power to heal is within you. It *is you*, literally. Directly accessing the Self is the first step on your healing journey and a greater quality of life. Through commanding your energies, you will be able to release/remove/destroy the disharmony at the root of all illness so that true repair and healing can occur. Anything short of this is merely treating symptoms. There is no magic pill, injection, or high-tech invention for true healing. Even if there were, we would learn very little to absolutely nothing about ourselves by having someone do it for us. (Plus, those side effects!) Waiting for others to fix or save us takes no accountability or responsibility. That is not the path of self-mastery. Authentic healers clear out disharmony that's currently occupying "space" within someone's consciousness and body of energies. The "patient" then reclaims themself. They simply move their awareness into the freedom and completeness of the Total Self, ending their experience of limitation, delusion, and disharmony.

We are perpetually responsible for ourselves on the grandest scale imaginable, even beyond the confines of space and time. When we abdicate any facet of our personal well-being to someone or something else, we stunt our individualized evolution, which is pointless because the very point of your existence is to know thy Self and all its infinite potential.

Instead of misidentifying with victimhood or waiting for something or someone to heal us, let's embrace our collective graduation into evolutionary adulthood. Empower yourself by taking full responsibility for enhancing the quality of your inner life. This empowerment disempowers the emotional, physical, and mental illnesses of the belief-based egoic identity and physical body. When we cease to *misidentify* with our imbalances, they will cease to have power over us. Our individual and collective consciousness is then raised in frequency, vibration, and awareness. This is ascension. And this is the higher purpose of the ATFHT.

Doing the work is the practice, and most of the steps in the healing technique are remarkably simple. Only the finite mind complicates and tries to interpret "what is" through logic and linearity, thus missing what "actually is." Empty your head of preconceived notions, knowledge, beliefs, and expectations. Forget what you have been told about what is possible and what isn't. If I would have listened to the well-meaning, highly knowledgeable, and compassionate health care practitioners regarding my own health, I'd still be in a wheelchair, most likely very ill, highly medicated, and quite possibly just a fading memory in the minds of some. Forget everything you think you know. Healing is not what you think it is. If it was, you would not still be in need of it. Instead, let's start fresh. An open mind and true humility are all you need to begin freeing yourself from the known (limitations).

The Modern-Day Magic of Intention and Imagination

First and foremost, true imagination—the infinite and omniscient Mind of Source/God/Creator—is the door to all possibilities. Everything starts with imagination when we embark on any journey, including the triumph of self-healing. Imagination is true magick. We are all powerful creators and ancient sorcerers. What people refer to as magick is simply working with higher frequential energy that is outside our physical sensory perceptions, which every one of us has the capacity to do based upon our individual level of Sentience. Throughout antiquity, there are countless stories of wizards, shamans, and mystics who worked with the Greater Reality by commanding unseen Intelligent Energy. Their work was referred to as magick because they were operating at frequencies outside our physical sensory perceptions and therefore prescribed mental comprehension. People didn't understand then and, for the most part, still don't know how it is done, so they termed it magick. We are going to demystify the mystery of true magick and alchemy.

Magick is actually a combination of enhanced access to the Total Self and the Greater Reality, and their higher functionality. When we access and direct higher frequential energy, we work with deeper aspects of the immortal Self and the Greater Reality, both of which exist outside our physical sensory perceptions. All true magick is done by accessing and manipulating higher frequential energy within ourselves and the Greater Reality. The way the energy is directed depends on our intention. It can be used for pure endeavors, like healing or accessing hidden wisdom to guide others, or for low-frequency ego-driven endeavors, including controlling or harming others. While these intentions and directed results have been labeled "white" magick and "black" magick, respectively, energy is just energy. It is the intention of the practitioner that gives it direction.

Demystifying the science of magick empowers and allows us to work toward becoming our very own version of Merlin the Great. The very real Merlin was an incarnation of a Timeless Master, and he utilized his immense wisdom, power, and abilities to bring about healing, change, and peace among all peoples. Merlin and other wizards were trained to use a variety of innate abilities, and just like us, they tended to be more skillful with some aspects of manipulating energy than with others. One of the fundamental steps in their training, though, was to learn how to use verbal commands. As you'll discover in step 7 of the ATFHT, incantations, mantras, and spells must be given the breath of life in order to affect the Greater Reality. That's why we "spell" words. They affect the energy within just as potently. What we say to ourselves and each other has great energetic impact. The depth and purity of our intention is the key to effectiveness. Our simultaneous surrender to the essence of the words' energetic intention takes its power to a whole other level.

While this may sound like fantasy, our intentions and words affect energy—and, therefore, what we call matter. One of the first people to demonstrate this in recent times was Dr. Masaru Emoto, whose extraordinary life work is documented in the *New York Times* bestseller *The Hidden Messages in Water*. His verifiable experiments demonstrated that thoughts, words, and sounds change the shape of water molecules. In one of the experiments, Emoto wrote an assortment of positive and negative words on bottles of distilled water. He froze the water and photographed it at subzero temperatures with a high-powered, microscopic camera. The water crystals in the bottles that had words such as *love, gratitude,* and *appreciation* written on them were symmetrical and resembled sacred geometry, with an iridescent quality. The water crystals from the bottles with words such as *hate* and *anger* written on them were asymmetrical and had dark holes in them. Similar experiments have been done using different frequency tones and their effect on the formation of sand. The takeaway from these experiments is being consciously aware of how our own thoughts and spoken words energetically affect us. This understanding is key in accruing greater self-awareness.

Sentience, through the power of intention, commands and greatly affects our own energy, and understanding this is a vital component of ascending the frequencies and self-healing. Therefore, our words can wield substantial power, and more obviously, so can our physical movements.

Performing specific gestures while reciting affirmations/mantras/spells can act as a multiplier by incorporating more of our energy field. Movement can be utilized to intensify the power of our intention. It can help us to feel more powerful, and therefore enhance the efficacy of the magick. Some practitioners, both historically and currently, use wands, staffs, or crystals as energy conductors. A wooden staff with a crystal attached to the business end with metal wiring can multiply kinetic intent. All of these elements—wood, base metals, and crystal—are excellent conductors of electricity. When done properly, they work synergistically as powerful multipliers of the directed energy/intention of the healing master. If your sentience directs you to work with a wand, staff, or crystal, go for it. But know that none of these tools are actually essential for healing. They are simply permission slips to command more of the Total Self and the Greater Reality. The highest level of alchemical magick and healing is performed simply through the use of pure and powerful intention. Working at the desire and intention frequencies, we are the most powerful, because these are higher, more potent frequencies than the thought, emotion, and physical frequential realms.

In order to access this Intelligent Energy, we must break free from body consciousness, see the limiting program of the belief-based egoic identity for what it is, and return to what we really are: formless, free, and unconditioned. This experiential knowing was the starting point for healing my toxic, diseased, and permanently paralyzed body, and you will use this same knowing to heal and free yourself.

Only Truth Frees and Heals You

Now that you know the fundamentals, we'll soon move on to step 1, where you can begin to recognize, deconstruct, and shed the belief-based egoic identity limitation program that runs by thinking. As you stop misidentifying sentience with the physical body and mental constructs, you can let go of all that is not original to you. Your life force returns and is now at your command. What remains, what is true, is divinity, perfection, and freedom.

In part 2 we're going to explore how real healing manifests and how to commandeer and work with Intelligent Energy. We will discover how to access higher-frequency states of consciousness that rejuvenate and repair and how to reprogram our misprogrammed energetic building blocks for optimal health. To aid our healing, we will first learn in the next chapter how to utilize the four directions of consciousness.

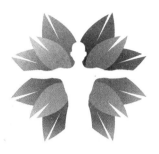

Chapter 3

Make Use of the Four Directions of Consciousness

To enhance the efficacy of the steps in the Ascend the Frequencies Healing Technique (ATFHT), it is extremely helpful for you to tangibly recognize which of the following directions of consciousness most resonates within you. Without realizing it, we perpetually utilize four essential avenues of consciousness during our life. Here are the four directions of consciousness:

1. Reason
2. Emotions and feelings
3. Faith
4. Will

We rely upon reason, emotions and feelings, faith, and our will for absolutely everything. In a nutshell, we mentally arrange data—the movement of the past—and use the intellect through deductive #1 reasoning. This is how we create our individual reality. We then take into account the weight of potential #2 emotions and feelings—born of misidentification with hierarchical belief systems—as it relates to our decision. Next, we utilize #3 faith in that we trust enough that the choice we have made is the way to go at that moment, which really equates to whatever is most in accordance with our hierarchical, belief-based egoic identity. Finally, we use our #4 will (energy)—normally at the behest of our egoic identity—to bring none, some, or all of it to fruition. There can be an omission or blend of all of these avenues, with some playing a bigger, lesser, or no role for each individual and each individual decision.

In my experience, these directions of consciousness are also what people utilize as the backdrop or contextual framework for their self-healing/personal development. What direction you choose is dependent on how you—the individualized sentience—prefer to work. You can utilize one or any combination of these four directions of consciousness to improve your health or any aspect of your life and to supercharge the ATFHT.

Notice how belief is not a true direction of consciousness. What's the difference between belief and faith? you may wonder. The gulf between the two is monumental.

Belief is anything whose landing spot lies outside of the Self. As an example, people say they believe in heaven, and it's somewhere out there, away from the Self. Belief, energetically speaking, is disempowering because it directs consciousness away from its source point within the Self. Faith, energetically speaking, is empowering because it provides the tangible experience deep within oneself. As an example, people say they feel God or the truth within their heart, within the Self. From a higher consciousness perspective, belief and faith are polar opposites.

I have worked with people who strongly resonate with a specific direction as well as some who are a hybrid. Personally, I utilized all of them to bring my Total Self into a single-pointedness of focus in order to manifest my "un-paralyzing."

Let's look at examples of how to utilize these four directions of consciousness.

1. Reason

Every vibrational wave of information within our body of energy has intelligence. The trillions of cells that comprise our "physical body" are replaced with new cells every seven years, which relates to the seven main chakras and seven main energetic templates that help create the human form. Therefore, it stands to reason that whatever is going on at this moment, our cells are perpetually working and designed to bring about harmony *if we allow them to*. Medical research has illustrated that liver cells live for only 150 days, and therefore every five months you have a new liver. You have a new heart every twenty years. A new lung every five months. A whole new skeleton every ten years. The entire surface layer of your skin is brand-new within four weeks. The cells in our intestines renew every five days. Our red blood cells are renewed within 120 days. Even our taste bud cells renew every two weeks.

Doesn't it stand to #1 reason that sickness is not a fixed state, considering the above?

The only constant is change, and you are the creator awareness of it. Do not believe in the reality of sickness, even when you are ill. Especially when you are ill. There is no valid reason to assume that what is momentarily going on in terms of your health is fixed or permanent. Nothing is. This is an example of how reason can be utilized to manifest a return to improved health.

2. Emotions and Feelings

Various states of emotion either defend us against ill health and promote healing or decrease our ability to ward off ill health and further promote disharmony and sickness.

When we are calm, at peace, and grateful, our attention resides within the Self. The Self is the bull's-eye and source point of our multi-frequential energy field. This is the optimum state of "beingness" for your highest quality of life and good health. When we are in our most harmonious state, mentally, emotionally, and physically, this balances our entire energy field and slows down the momentum of any disharmony and decrepitude. Disharmony cannot grow within a harmonious environment.

In general, emotions are of a lower frequency (existing in the human realm) and feelings are of a higher frequency (existing in the purely energetic realms).

When we are in any state of emotional or mental extreme, specifically one that causes a contraction (exclusiveness) rather than an expansion (inclusiveness) of our energy field, we no longer reside in the bull's-eye of our energy field's optimal harmonious state. This creates a disharmonious current or wave of energy that then permeates our entire physical body and ultimately leads to ill health.

The processing or non-suppression of emotions tends to create a dualistic experience created by the false "I." Rather than seeing emotions as something to process and work through, see them as bad code or misinformation that is simply being identified with by your lower consciousness because it's in your field of non-self-awareness. Emotions run and are interpreted by your egoic mind. Your false identity must already be present and in control of your consciousness in order for the emotional imbalance to even make itself known. Instead of processing emotions or worrying about not suppressing them, realize they are simply something that passes through your field of lower awareness and body of energy. They have no real correlation or connection to the Self. Therefore, don't analyze, ignore, or suppress them; just let them be, don't indulge them, and they will be alchemized by the supreme vibration of the Self.

The harboring of negative thoughts and emotions is a contraction of energy. This contraction is a function and by-product of the false self. Our low-frequency belief-based egoic identity only conflates the human misperceptions, misunderstandings, and misidentifications of who we think we are and how we feel about ourselves. Subsequently, this is how we view, interact with, and relate to ourselves and the outside world: through massive limitations. Misidentifying with thoughts, emotions, the body, and experiences the body has literally embeds them within our body of energy. Subsequently, we cause the imbalance and erosion of our originally balanced personal multi-frequential energy field. In turn, the physical body then encodes these misidentifications by running their misprogramming through the experience of disharmony, disease, decrepitude, and demise.

If misidentification with beliefs, concepts, thoughts, emotions, physicality, and experiences is thorough enough, the sentience and body of energy we work with will carry these misidentifications around with them wherever the sentience goes, including other incarnations. This can lead to birth abnormalities or defects outside of our inherited genetic lineage.

By working with the unencumbered Total Self directly, which we discovered in step 1, embedded misperceptions, misunderstandings, and misidentifications come to the conscious surface because they are a product of the egoic identity. By utilizing step 1, these limitation programs are no longer running, because the false "I" is no longer holding our consciousness and energy captive. Instead, we tangibly realize our true essence. Now our old attachments and misidentifications can be consciously recognized, removed, or dissolved through the rest of the steps.

Laughter is a tremendous boost to the immune system and works immediately on the release of free radicals within our energy field. Laughter produces a vibratory state that is of higher frequency. This higher frequency "shakes loose" all of the information that has become stuck within our energy field. Laughter is also a really fun way to self-heal. Only the egoic identity, with its limiting body consciousness, takes itself and things seriously. Sentience has no desire to control a single thing. Instead, it tangibly experiences its own limitless depth and imagination through endless creativity.

Chatting with a friend or family member who makes you truly laugh or watching a video that you genuinely find hysterical is extremely beneficial to your healing. Deep belly laughs are tremendously effective in raising your vibration. As a healing practice, try spending at least an hour of your daily life without a care in the world by experiencing authentic heartfelt laughter and joy.

Self-deprecating humor is also extremely cathartic, as it exposes the hang-ups and misperceptions that the egoic identity has about itself. Laughter truly is one of the best medicines, and sharing a laugh brings us all closer together. Laughter has tremendous transformative powers. Personally, I laughed all the time during my healing journey, and still do. I never took my temporary body's situation seriously by misidentifying with it, so it had no real power over me. My unwavering focus and complete dedication to my challenges were ever present, and so was my sense of humor about it.

While I was in my hospital bed, the physical therapists would have me use leg loops because of my chest-down paralysis. Leg loops are long, stretchy bands I used to "lasso" my legs in order to bring my feet and legs up to me. It was the only way I could put on my shoes, socks, underwear, shorts, etc. Part of my therapy included the monitoring of my daily progress to make sure I would be able to dress myself once I was discharged. One day, while in my hospital bed utilizing the leg loops, I accidentally dropped my sneaker onto the floor. When you're paralyzed from the chest down and in bed, getting anything off the floor can be quite an ordeal, if not downright impossible. After dropping my sneaker, I said to the physical therapists, "Don't worry. I'll get it. It's not like I'm paralyzed." We all laughed. Hard. I never misidentified my immortal Self with bodily paralysis and therefore never took it seriously. It's part of why I transcended all temporary limitations.

Gratitude, which is being thankful for what is, is a powerful and harmonizing energetic state. As a practice, take a moment and realize the immense fullness of every single now by simply being totally present. Surrender any personal agenda or self-judgment. Tangibly realize that every now is literally a miracle of sublime creation and this is how you are meant to live, as an expression of this. Do this repeatedly throughout the day until this state of being becomes normalized.

Dedication to the practice of gratitude can lead one into a state of pure grace. Grace is the conscious awareness of the gift of the human experience bestowed upon us in order to expedite the accrual of sentience. This life is truly a blessing and a gift, and like all gifts, they are best when shared. It is an opportunity to express our divinity within physical reality. Grace in action is to be in compassionate service to your own life plan while simultaneously in service to others, sans any egoic gratification. Showing gratitude for the very opportunity to experience physical life can be utilized to raise one's frequency, which repairs and harmonizes the lower-frequency misprogramming of the egoic identity. Gratitude enhances the quality of all life in ways that are not even calculable.

Gratitude is an example of a feeling rather than an emotion.

3. Faith

Complete and total faith elevates you past the belief-based egoic identity limitation program. Faith puts your consciousness in direct connection to the Source of life within *you*. It exists prior to and therefore transcends any transient belief-based program of limitations and its conceptualized, fragmentary concept of what a life is or should be. Faith imbues the physical plane with the love and power of divinity through our direct connection with Self. Those with true faith can and have experienced instantaneous "healing" because they are working with the creator Self directly. Those who experience authentic spontaneous healing do so because it is in their life plan. When we truly know within the depths of our being, not our body/mind complex, we have true faith. Some people resonate with this direction or avenue of consciousness and therefore utilize it to initiate, enhance, and accelerate their recovery or transcendence from disharmony and a poor quality of life. Healers, too, can work directly through this preferred direction of consciousness.

When we connect to true faith, we connect directly to the origination of the cosmos itself—the One Self—and all of its infinite possibilities, which include transcending ill health. When physical, emotional, mental, or purely energetic healing manifests, it is tangible proof that you have transcended the current challenge in your energy field. Bravo!

Faith is a powerful direction of consciousness that can be harnessed and utilized by anyone for the purpose of improved quality of life and health. Faith is not a mental, emotional, or physical exercise but rather a direct experiential knowingness of the divine within you. This is an aspect of gnosis. I knew, deep within my Self, that total faith was intrinsic to transcending the permanent paralysis and life-threatening conditions. To have true faith, we must surrender in totality. This is the ultimate display of courage and trust. To do that, the belief-based egoic identity must no longer have control.

We may have heard or even said the prayer, "Father, thy will, not mine, be done." Our life plan, our soul's purpose, is God's will. The two are one and the same. When you work in complete accordance with your life plan, you are compelled. This is faith in action. Free will is what we have already planned for ourselves, oddly enough.

"Mighty Spirit, thy will, not mine, be done" is the only prayer I said while in the hospital. The total surrender empowered me beyond comprehension. That statement may seem like a paradox, but the experiential reality of it is anything but that. Do it and see for yourself what happens.

4. Will

The will is the harnessing of your body of energy. Once your intention is unwavering and permanently fixed, your will becomes the road map your life force follows in order to bring your destiny into reality. The complete and total union of your sentience and your complement of energy translates into your divine will (true energetic power).

Strengthening of the will comes from never breaking your intention. Now you are working with your willpower. The train of unbroken intention is a powerhouse of energy roaring at high speed along the tracks of your nervous system. Intention is what keeps you headed on a direct and nonstop trip to the destination of your desire. When you entertain doubt, you send a contradictory electric current that breaks your original electric current. Now you have to start all over again. The moment you doubt that you will arrive at your intended destination, the train—now powered by the energy of doubt—has to jump tracks onto wherever the doubtful mind track has shifted to. Where attention goes, your energy flows. You will never arrive at the intended location of your highest desire if you keep switching destinations by jumping onto the tracks of doubt.

Doubt must be removed even as a mere possibility. If you doubt your victory, ask yourself, "Who is it that doubts?" The answer will be "Me. I am the one who doubts it." Then simply ask yourself, "Who am I?" The mind will go blank because that who is an illusion. That who is your limitation program running. Pay no attention to the petulant child we call the egoic identity. The most potent use of willpower occurs when you have freed your focus and attention from the tyranny of your program of limitations. Marry your focus with your will so that they become one. Now absolutely nothing can break your spirit. Ever. This is being *invincible*. The complete mastery over your energetic power is your indomitable will in action. It is your destiny as an immortal, limitless creator being.

You will feel immense power when working at the highest potentiality of your will. Anyone who has ever truly pushed themselves past their prescribed false limitations knows precisely what this feels like. Nothing seems impossible, because at this level, *nothing is*. Inevitability walks in step with your indomitable will. At what moment your physical, emotional, mental, or energetic healing becomes totally manifest is irrelevant, because you are repairing yourself now. It is already happening. You are "willing" yourself to heal. Fully accept your healing. The voice in your head who refuses to accept it or is simply too impatient isn't you.

✻ ✻ ✻

To bring life back into my paralyzed and toxic body, I utilized reason, feelings/emotions, and faith to a single-pointedness of focus. I fully activated this single-pointedness with the harnessing of my indomitable will to heal myself, along with a complete detachment from any future result.

I would bring all of my focus to the present moment. Complete inner stillness and silence. This allowed me to regain control over my entire complement of life force energy. With supreme focus and fervent desire, I would verbalize the command "I bring life into my spine and legs now." As I did this, simultaneously I would remember exactly what it felt like to have full sensation from the chest down and precisely what it felt like to walk. This would make the electrical signals of powerful intention reignite throughout my damaged nervous system. I had to rebuild those damaged tracks. While fully committed to the above, I would either have my legs manually manipulated to simulate the walking motion or manipulate them myself using leg loops while lying down. This supreme and heartfelt focus allowed me to exist in a perpetual state of powerful higher consciousness creativity. Past and future did not exist because my attention wasn't on anything other than the process of transformation.

I sent absolutely no contradictory electrical impulses of doubt. Not one, ever. (You'll learn in step 1 how to counter these unhelpful thoughts.) I harnessed all my energy into the healing of my paralyzed body. All of it. In this sense, I simply willed myself to walk again. I was not going to be denied my victory, and yet I was at total peace. My will was complete, resolute, unbreakable…invincible. The mastery over my physical form was simply a matter of complete control over my energy into a single-pointedness. Embodying both an iron will and complete detachment allowed me to harness what I always knew in my heart into experiential reality…the victory of transcendence! Do the same for your Self.

The Self's Preferred Healing Avenue

You can utilize one or any combination of these four directions of consciousness to greatly improve your quality of life and to super-charge your steps of the ATFHT. In order to determine which one most resonates with you personally, let's inquire within.

As you look at the four directions of consciousness—(1) reason, (2) emotions and feelings, (3) faith, and (4) will—ask yourself which direction intuitively resonates with you. If nothing immediately jumps out at you, that's okay. Simply complete the following sentence:

I tend to experience my best results when I ...

1. use my head.
2. trust my gut feeling.
3. know that I am being guided.
4. use my determination.

Once you recognize which way best suits you, merge yourself with it by no longer second-guessing your decision. Trust your Self. All of these avenues work perfectly; it's simply a matter of personal preference in terms of how you work best.

We now understand that what we really are is sentience that is given energy to create with. It is only our egoic identity formed from limitations that stifles our imagination. This program of misperceptions, misunderstandings, and misidentifications leaves us woefully disempowered. This inhibits our innate ability to properly command and direct our own self-healing. With the discovery of which avenue of consciousness most resonates within us, we are properly positioned to begin the reclaiming of our own well-being. Now, we can begin, with true power and pristine clarity, the revolutionary ATFHT.

Part 2

Ascend the Frequencies Healing Technique (ATFHT)

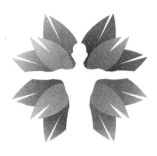

Step 1

Access Your True Essence

Who or, more accurately, *what* is the real you?

In part 1, we established that we're not our physical body, and we're also not our EMI, or egoic identity, which is the conceptualized character we create with whom we misidentify our immortal Self. While this is a simple truth, the finite human mind will do its best to stop you from embracing it. Nonacceptance is how the belief-based egoic identity protects itself from demise, because self-awareness exposes the false self for the parasite that it is. The finite and conditioned human mind is separation, division, compartmentalization, and memorization. It does this endlessly, with everything, including to itself, through nonstop analysis and judgment. It operates more like a parasitical virus, trying to divide, conquer, and subdue its host. It perpetually separates and therefore can never see unity when it looks within or at the world. Your egoic identity is disharmony itself and can only produce further disharmony. It woefully lacks any authentic power, and it's why we cannot heal ourselves or evolve our sentience while in servitude to it.

Like a computer virus, your limitation program is always running as your default setting—but you can override it.

Sentience—what we really are—is always aware. It commands energy into your mental body, which produces the phenomenon called thinking. Thinking is simply the movement of the past. One cannot be the awareness of thoughts and the victim of them at the same time. That is simply impossible. What actually happens is we lose the Self through misidentification with the creation of thought. Your egoic identity reaches for thoughts and other sensory stimuli simply to perpetuate and reinforce its sense of a separate self. This is why inner stillness and silence is death for the egoic identity. Stillness within stops your program of limitations from running. Without thought, your belief-based egoic identity ceases to run its program. Without belief, there is no thinking, for belief is the context for all thought. Without thought, your limitation program ceases to run. What remains is tangibly true: freedom, limitless imagination, and joy!

There is nothing inherent within awareness itself that implies ownership of what awareness perceives. Ownership is a concept and, like all concepts, is just an illusion. All concepts are a mental fragment or reduction of the oneness of existence. This is what the finite human mind does. It separates, fragments, compartmentalizes, and divides. Thought is a delusion ripped from the unity of all existence.

You choose your feelings just as you choose your thoughts. You may not consciously be aware of this because of your deep programming born of the reactionary state of your belief-based egoic identity. Think of it this way: the belief-based egoic identity judges and reacts, while sentience observes and responds. The egoic identity must react because it misidentifies itself with the experience. Hence, we become a victim to our creations as well as other people's creations. This is why you may struggle with control of emotions. This also provides a glimpse into how disharmony manifests within our body of originally pure energy.

Sometimes you choose to watch a scary movie so you can experience the thrills and chills. But if you just observed the movie in a detached state, you would never get scared by what's on the screen. You could choose to read a romantic novel to experience passion and desire. You choose the feeling you want to experience by what you reach for, but you eternally remain the awareness of it all. And just like thoughts, because you are aware of feelings, you cannot "be" your feelings. You are the sentient awareness that commands the energy within your larger body of energy in order to experience these temporary creations. You are always aware of what you feel, which also makes "being" the feeling impossible. Thinking that you are the feeling is also a product of deep-rooted misidentification. Just like thoughts, if you were your feelings, when they pass you would pass too. Yet you remain right here, with me, right now.

Let's look at the monumental gulf between "being" and "identifying." For example, when I say "I love drumming," I instantly connect with the feeling of unlimited creative musical expression, the joy of a rhythm that flows through my entire being, and the internal freedom I experience when I'm open to inspiration. It's pure joy, and time literally ceases to exist.

In comparison, when I say "I am a drummer," I immediately feel the weight and responsibility of what "being a drummer" means to me as a belief or concept. A previous mental and emotional place-holder now has to be lived up to: Am I good enough to call myself a drummer? Shouldn't I be able to make money from playing? Will other people think I'm good enough to call myself a drummer? Shouldn't I know more patterns, techniques, and time sequences?

The moment I misidentify myself as a drummer, joy and freedom are replaced with the conceptualized mental responsibility and emotional weight associated with the concept of what it means to me when I say "I am a drummer." While "I love drumming" and "I'm a drummer" seem similar, they are the difference between freedom, joy, and unlimited creative expression and the onerous, confining responsibility of a role. Transitioning from "being" to "identifying" happens nearly instantaneously due to the control your egoic identity has over your beingness. Detachment or pure observation is required to tangibly and experientially know the difference.

Identification suffocates imagination. It enslaves your sentience, imprisoning its freedom and supernatural ability to endlessly create harmonic perfection in a limitless fashion. Once incarnate, your primary creation born of misidentification, the egoic identity, is the entire cause of your suffering. What you really are is simply too large, limitless, perfect, and divine to fit into the totality of all beliefs, concepts, and ideologies.

Many of my students quickly grasp that they are not their thoughts but struggle with emotions. Many say, "I can't help but feel how I feel." For now, you cannot help how you feel because it's part of the limitation program of who you think you are and how you feel about yourself. This is how the egoic identity works. Remember, you are the awareness of everything, not what you are the awareness of.

The egoic identity creates and experiences life through a conglomeration of past stimuli that you misidentify as the Self. All sensory phenomena, even the physical body, are transient and eventually disappear. Mistakenly, you identify with these transitory phenomena and believe in their authenticity and permanence. This disharmony leads to all disease and disrepair, because all disharmony is created through disharmonious thought patterns. Your ability to perceive beliefs, thoughts, emotions, the body, and its experiences means they're not you. They are projections, while you—sentience—are a pristine creator and the awareness of it all.

Sentience gives depth, context, and understanding to every single moment of your entire existence, incarnate or not. In truth, we're observing our "human experience" when we play with our pets, talk with our friends, go out to dinner, or play an instrument. Otherwise, without our perpetual observation, how would we know that anything is taking place? You are not the thought, feeling, action, hope, expectation, belief, body, or egoic identity. Therefore, you're not who you *think* you are or how you feel about yourself. You're way beyond all of that. Sentience is immortal creator awareness given energy to work with. Sentience has the desire to know and evolve itself. The human experience is simply one way sentience accrues and deepens.

Once a belief-based, habitual mental construct of who we think we are and how we feel about ourselves has been formed, we run this limitation program with every stimulus, including people, we encounter thereafter. That program runs by thinking.

For example, when information (sensory-perceived data) is aligned with our belief-based programming, we welcome it onboard and work with it. When somebody expresses an opinion that backs up a belief you identify with, like when you hear that someone you already don't like did something bad that you didn't know about, you then use this new information as confirmation bias, or proof that your belief is true. Similarly, when information doesn't coincide with facets of our programming, we reject it and often get "triggered." Maybe that same person whom you hold a negative belief about just did something considered kind. That new information will cause cognitive dissonance, because it doesn't coincide with your programming (beliefs). One or the other must then be rejected. Either way, you are trapped within duality. Thought comes from beliefs and is filtered through the egoic identity, while inspiration is born directly of Sentience. This direct alignment with the Sentience is what is known as "being in the zone." Ideas are flowing to the person without any filtering, critiquing, or other mental interference. A new solution for any problem or challenge is an example of this.

The identity is the ego. The ego is the mind. The mind is thought itself, and thought is simply the movement of the past (fed by beliefs/concepts/ideologies). Thinking is the past. Even if we imagine a future, it is always based upon the past. There is no self-healing when one dwells in the past or projects it into the future. All your power is in reclaiming the energy your egoic identity has hijacked. This occurs while fully experiencing the freedom and limitlessness built into every moment. The egoic identity is simply a construct that continually pushes the limitations of the past forward rather than experiencing the only reality that authentically exists: now, "what is." Fresh, infinite possibilities.

The Limitations of So-Called Knowledge

So-called knowledge is a collection of justified beliefs. It's the accumulation of information from our senses that we're capable of parroting in order to perform some task that is bound by time. All human endeavors are always bound by time. Anything that we learn falls under this umbrella. For example, we memorize the alphabet in order to form words so we can communicate via the written word or speech. This is necessary and certainly fits the criteria above. Once we leave the physical plane, it is of no use, and therefore was bound by time. Telepathy is then utilized and is a far more expressive and illuminating form of communication.

How about learning to become an acupuncturist? You memorize the information and then mimic it through repetition. Here are the meridians of the body, here's where we're supposed to place the needles, etc. Knowledge is just imitation and repetition of the past based upon justified beliefs. All so-called knowledge, no matter the subject, works in this fashion. Metaphysically speaking, so-called knowledge is beneath your true wisdom and limitless imagination.

In essence, this so-called knowledge is a lot like the egoic identity: belief in its authenticity, programmed acceptance, misidentification, and imitation followed by adherence through repetition. As previously stated, all knowledge is the past. And the same holds true for beliefs, concepts, ideologies, and philosophies. They are all projections of the finite, transient egoic identity. Conditioning, really. Programming.

The egoic identity has no direct connection with unconditional love or timeless wisdom. It's no wonder that our miscreated, limited, temporary, delusional identities cannot heal ourselves or each other. It's also no wonder true happiness, unconditional love, compassion, and joy are in such rare supply.

Sentience—What We Really Are— Resides Between Our Heart and Spine

Have you ever noticed when we want to indicate ourselves to someone, we always tap the center of our chest and say "me"? Nobody ever points to their head. Interesting, right? It's because our *sentience*—what we really are—resides in the center of our chest between the heart and spine.

Our energy source, which is not the same as sentience, resides a bit lower in the body, closer to kidney level, just below the belly button and above the groin. Sentience commands energy. I'm going to teach you how to properly access and utilize your sentience and energy to repair, heal, and greatly improve the quality of your life. These protocols are the exact ones I used to heal from chronic disease, life-threatening ailments, and "permanent" chest-down paralysis. None of this would have been possible if I had bought into the justified beliefs accepted as so-called medical knowledge. What is required for you, too, to achieve the "impossible" is simply your transcendence of the limiting delusions of your belief-based egoic identity and its low-frequency body consciousness. The longer we identify with anything, the greater disharmony we create within ourselves. We are formless, free, and unconditioned. Our only bondage is not tangibly realizing this.

Step 1 Shortcuts to Dissolve the Ego/Mind/Identity

These practices will act as shortcuts to help you dial down the ego mind. They will help you to drop away from your beliefs and instead enter into your natural harmonious state. Part of this practice involves self-inquiry. Self-inquiry is a direct and powerful way to dissolve what has gotten in the way of the Self. When the fire of self-inquiry is burning, stoke that flame. It will burn away everything that you are not. In the beginning, do the following four exercises as outlined precisely here: (1) Ask Yourself, "Who Am I?" (2) Fingers to Chest, (3) Imagine You're a Pair of Eyes Floating in Space, and (4) Say "I Don't Know." Do each exercise for five minutes, individually, three separate times a day: once upon waking, once before lunch, and again before dinner or going to sleep. These protocols are effortless; increase your usage as much as you like.

Ask Yourself, "Who Am I?"

Whenever you have a thought, any thought, ask yourself, "To whom has this thought arisen?"

The answer will be: "To me. I am the one having this thought."

Then ask yourself, "Who am I?"

The mind will go blank because there is no "who." That "who" is the belief-based ego identity, a parasite. Ultimately, there is but one spirit moving through all of existence: Source/God/Creator.

The continued practice of "Who am I?" will eventually dissolve the nagging questioner, the reactionary voice inside your head. That unloving and wholly judgmental presence is the originator and source of your suffering.

The belief-based egoic identity is a temporary delusion that must be seen clearly to be shed. It is the source of all suffering.

The repeated practice of "Who am I?" will eventually allow our individual attention to dwell directly within its source, or origin, which is our sentience. Once there, dwell within that space. There is no need to leave or operate outside of the direct connection with what you really are. The best of yourself, the highest quality of life, is contingent upon your ability to stay here. Remember, our sentience resides in the center of the chest between the heart and spine. With every moment that our attention is upon and within this infinite stillness and all-encompassing silence, our body of energy begins to harmonize and repair itself. Like a balloon on a string, when we let go of the egoic identity, its misprogramming, which creates ill health, begins to float away. By practicing self-inquiry, we continually place our attention on the Source within, which is our sentience, and we experience peace and harmony. Now what is deeply embedded within our body of energy can be worked with, repaired, and healed.

Stay in this state of pure self-awareness not through force but with a gentle tenacity. When another thought or emotion pops up, simply repeat the practice of self-inquiry. Ask yourself, "To whom has this thought or emotion arisen?" Your answer will be "to me."

Ask yourself, "Who am I?" Keep doing this until it has become normalized to dwell within the empty space or no-mind state. Delicately harness your intention to surrender. It's not as hard you may "think." It's no different than setting a cup on a table and knowing it will remain there without you exerting force to keep it there. You let it rest where it's been placed. There's no effort involved. All the effort and straining is in reaching for and holding the cup.

Carrying around luggage all day is exhausting and straining, but putting it down is effortless. Do the same with the egoic identity. Don't worry—all of its mental, emotional, physical, and energetic baggage will be there waiting for you. If you want all that suffering back, simply pick the beliefs back up. Or you can leave them here with me and free yourself. It's up to you.

If you feel upset, ask yourself, "Who is it that is upset?" *Me.* "Who am I?" The emotion will fade away because the creator of the emotion, your belief-based egoic identity, is not getting any energy to sustain it. If you get anxious, ask yourself, "Who is it that feels anxious?" *Me.* "Who am I?" You will instantly become calmer. If you're afraid, ask, "Who is it that's afraid?" *Me.* "Who am I?" Your programming will dissolve, and along with it, its fear. The belief-based egoic identity is the fight-or-flight reactionary state. It's why, eventually, everyone gets sick, suffers, and dies. Something so riddled with disharmony—namely, our body of energy and its physical component—eventually becomes incapable of housing such divinity and perfection (sentience). Do this self-inquiry practice until the mind and body knows its place. Likewise, physical discomfort and pain will have less of a hold over you when you ask, "Who is it that feels pain?" *I do.* "Who am I?"

We can begin to manage our physical discomfort much better once we stop misidentifying with the "experiencer" of the sensation, the physical body. We remain as awareness of the sensation of pain instead of identifying with the "experiencer" of the pain or the pain itself. The human form is simply the conduit or vehicle for sentience to experience physical reality. This includes the sensations of both pain and pleasure. There must be recognition of the truth that we are not the body/mind nor their sensations/perceptions in order to transcend these experiences. We cannot transcend what we drag around as the false "I."

Let Go of Baggage (Past, Future, and Thought)
Imagine my voice guiding you as you read the following:

- Sit in a relaxed position, with your feet firmly planted on the floor, eyes closed, palms up while resting on the uppermost part of your thighs.

- Inhale through the nose and exhale out the mouth, utilizing the diaphragm. Take three very deep breaths and completely empty the lungs and diaphragm on the exhale.

- Imagine that you just bought a lot of groceries. Your grocery bags are filled to the brim, and when you pick them up, you feel how heavy they are. It's straining your arms and your back to carry these groceries to your car. Feel how taxing it is to exert yourself like this. Feel the strain and tension in your face, neck, and shoulders. Your arms and hands are stressed by holding on to these heavy bags. Your lower back and stomach tighten. Your legs and feet also feel the additional burden. Your mind is overloaded trying to manage this level of exertion and strain. You know you can't carry these groceries around much longer. It's painful and exhausting.

- Now imagine what it feels like when you simply put the groceries down. Just let go of the bags. Leave them. They will be there later if you want them. Just let go. Feel how light and unstressed your body feels again. Feel the unburdened physical nature of a clear mind. Feel how you are no longer worried and how your body isn't stressed now that you aren't carrying all of those groceries around with you.

- Now do the same with all of your past thoughts, feelings, and experiences. Just let them go like so many groceries you have been carrying around. They are not you. Just let them all go. Unburden yourself fully. You have permission to let the past drop to the ground. Leave it all at *my* feet. I will take care of it for you.

- Now do the same with your future expectations. Just let them go. Unburden yourself completely. You have permission to do so. Let them drop to the ground. Leave all of those at *my* feet too. I will take care of them for you.

- Stay here, totally unencumbered with me. Free. Free from the past or future. There is no need to ever pick them up again. I will take care of them for you.

- Forgive yourself for thinking these burdens were yours to carry. Forgive others who mistakenly agreed with you and thought they were yours to bear as well.

There's no need to pick up anything ever again. I will take care of it for you. Just be your perfect free Self, now, from this moment on.

Fingers to Chest

Using one of your hands, gently touch the tips of your index and middle fingers directly to the center of your chest. Feel the soft pressure of your fingers there. Bring all of your attention and focus to the sensation of touch in the center of your chest. Remain right there without analyzing. You will immediately find that it's difficult to think or emote. Stay there. Now, from inside the center of your chest, gently reach out and touch your fingertips. This fully opens your heart chakra, which activates your direct reunion with the Self—sentience. Keep all of your attention and focus there, in the center of your chest. You may instantaneously experience peace, an undercurrent of joy, almost like laughter, a state of no mind, total clarity, great power, and a sense of completeness. That's the real you! Just stay there. You're experiencing the absence of the disharmonious filter of the belief-based egoic identity running its limitation program called thinking.

This presence in the center of your chest is the Real You—sentience. The immortal, divine, and limitless You is right there between your heart and spine. Sentience is the pure creator awareness. At this moment, you are free from misprogramming. The physical body begins to repair itself in this natural harmonious state. When your belief-based egoic identity ceases to run its program of limitations, self-healing begins. A far greater power and enhanced quality of life is experienced.

Imagine You're a Pair of Eyes Floating in Space

Once you have settled into the Self using self-inquiry or the fingers to the chest, imagine yourself as just your physical eyes floating in space with no connection to the brain. Just pure creator awareness and its innate freedom. Objective nonanalytic perception. The tangible experiential seeing of "what is" not filtered through belief-based judgment. Your depth of wisdom, understanding, and compassion are built into the very fabric of your pure "floating eyes."

When you practice this exercise, you may feel a surge of joy because your energy drops down from your lower astral, mental, and emotional bodies. This is normal because you are no longer giving the egoic identity any attention. Floating eyes promote the tangible recognition of your sentience in the center of your chest. Again, stay there. Recognize and feel the presence within. Don't analyze anything. Without the disharmonious egoic identity, there are no thoughts to obscure your connectivity to all life, divine intelligence, and higher frequency. That is because our attention is now directly within the bull's-eye of the Self. Now our natural energetic defenses are at their strongest, because we have reclaimed our body of energy. We can think of the concentric rings that encircle the bull's-eye as your multi-frequential auric layers being properly filled with energetic life force. This acts as a natural barrier against all free radicals (information) that can potentially harm your energy field.

You begin to repair your body of energy just by doing this. Repair and defense happen naturally, because being centered is our natural harmonious state. Think of it this way: our entire multi-frequential body of energy, including the physical, is most robust at warding off illness when it is attuned directly to the Self.

Say "I Don't Know"

Ask yourself a question you don't know the answer to and don't care about. The fastest way to clear your lower astral and mental body of information is to simply ask yourself a question that you genuinely don't know the answer to. Make it a question where you have absolutely no clue, not even a good guess, as to the answer. It is also important not to have any real interest in the answer as well. Here are some example questions to ask yourself:

- How many hairs are on a cat?
- How many windows are there in New York City?
- How many stop signs are there in all of Eastern Europe?

The answer to all of them is "I don't know and I don't care." The "I don't know and I don't care" state empties our lower astral, mental, and emotional container. It clears our thoughts, memories, and expectations, which, in effect, hits the pause button on the disharmonious egoic identity limitation program.

Let your energy naturally drop down and return to its Source point within the physical body, located just below the belly button and above the groin.

Clear Old Disharmonious Thought Patterns

When the egoic identity has been disempowered, mental constructs are replaced with your innate completeness and the freedom of imagination. Your thought process then changes. This alters the emotions you experience, the actions you take, the experiences you reach out for, and the behaviors you adopt. This is tangible proof of your healing, greater quality of life, and awakening. This and the following shortcut

exercise will help you to clear yourself of old disharmonious beliefs/
concepts, which provide the context for thoughts, emotions, actions,
and behaviors.

- When a thought pops into your head, do not grab hold of it
  and ruminate on it.
- Observe the thought from a neutral perspective.
- Do not formulate a relationship with the thought by indulg-
  ing in it.
- Observe the thought floating away like a helium-filled balloon when you let go of the string of identification. Don't
  try to grab for the thought.
- Repeat as needed.

Clear Old Disharmonious Emotional Patterns

- When a disharmonious emotion enters your energetic field,
  do not identify with it or indulge in it.
- Observe the emotion from a neutral perspective, like you
  would watch a breeze billowing the curtains on a window.
- Do not formulate a relationship with the emotion by analyzing it. That analysis will become the problem itself and
  will then require answers. This is simply a self-perpetuating
  downward spiral of energy.
- Imagine yourself being completely hollow, like a balloon, and
  simply observe the emotion pass right through the empty
  porous membrane of the balloon.
- Repeat as needed.

❄ ❄ ❄

Once we stop the belief-based program of limitations from running, we regain our energy. This affords the experience of peace,
clarity, harmony, and connectivity to the Self. Your indomitable power

resides within harnessing the Total Self. Return to the bull's-eye center point within your energy field.

We don't need to, nor should we, endlessly think about everything. It's a complete misuse and abuse of our life force. Our energy, through gentle intention, must be redirected to its source so the egoic identity stops creating disharmony for our body of energy. Remember, wisdom and compassion flow through our consciousness on the river of intuition—not through thinking. The only impediment to this eternal and divine flow is the energetic thievery at the behest of your belief-based false self and its incessant ruminations.

When we physically lie down, we stop using our intention, which is the current of energy we send to our nerves that contracts the muscles around our skeleton in order to support our body. When we lie down, we give ourselves permission to relax, repair, and rejuvenate. Do the same with your egoic identity. Through intention, allow your sentience and energy to return to its source within you. Do not underestimate the incredible transformative powers of the protocols in step 1: (1) Ask Yourself, "Who Am I?" (2) Fingers to Chest, (3) Imagine You're a Pair of Eyes Floating in Space, and (4) Say "I Don't Know." They dissolve the habitual and ritualistic machinations of your disharmonious programming.

My clients and students report that they have never felt freer, more peaceful, less stressed, and more joyful using these protocols. They also report less pain and an unwavering feeling of self-empowerment. Consequently, they began a return to better health simply by performing these four exercises. That is because they had their energy back. This is direct transformation and goes beyond mere change. Change implies the residue of the past, while transformation creates something new. This is what neuroplasticity, or the rewiring of the brain, attempts to achieve. Now we are doing it for our entire body of multi-frequential energy. By working directly, consciously, with the Self, we achieve the ultimate in repair, self-healing, and a far greater quality of life because we go to what is original to each of us…the perfect completeness of total freedom.

The Importance of Being in the Meditative State for Self-Healing

All of the steps in this program make use of the meditative state, and this is important. When alone in my hospital room, which was roughly eighteen to nineteen hours of the day, I was in communion with powerful self-healing in what could loosely be described as a perpetual higher-consciousness meditative state. I want to be clear about what I mean when I talk about meditation: total peace, clarity, connectivity, communion, enhanced functionality of higher intuitive functions, gratitude, and an absence of thoughts and identifications. All of this may seem strange, but it's true nonetheless. In order for thoughts to ever occur, there must be an active egoic identity already present.

The Self is meditation. You are what exists before thought. Meditation—the Self—is the most powerful way to transcend your egoic program of limitations. To experience and maintain a heightened level of connectivity, calmness, communion, and clarity, you must go well beyond the realm of the physical body's outwardly focused, limited physical senses and its resultant finite intellect. In other words, in order to perceive the limitless and divine, one must be in a limitless and divine state. Meditation reveals what is—the omniscient higher mind of Source and its limitless imagination expressing itself within you, as you, *now*.

Our wisdom, love, and power are automatically activated within the action of pure observation, not analysis. This is meditation. It is the awakening of our divine intelligence. Focusing on anything while meditating is not meditating at all. That is exclusion, which occurs through contraction. The direct, experiential knowingness of the impermanence of this lifetime and our nonidentification with anything contained within it is meditation.

Your egoic identity and its limited body consciousness are the debilitating anchors you addictively imprison your immortal consciousness with, and this prevents true meditation and liberation from personhood. But you can change this! Being free of your program of limitations and any misidentifications is the *starting line* to the awakening of cosmic consciousness, not the finish line. Being free of misidentification is the moment you are truly born. This is meditation. You are no longer bound by limitations.

The concept of lack is the realm of the unawakened mind—the limited egoic identity and body consciousness—while meditation is the abundance of here and now. Meditation is clarity, calmness, communion, and connectivity—where the illusionary, transient program of limitations and all its projections evaporate. The meditative state does not lack anything nor desire anything, as sentient awareness is self-sustaining and eternally complete. When you live this way, you liberate and transcend the limited ego mind, which anchors your infinite imagination. Complete detachment from the mental prison of the ego mind, of thought itself, is the liberation of meditation.

Of course, most people "think" they do not have the so-called luxury of being in a constant meditative state. We have jobs, families, things to do, places to go, etc. But the opposite is actually true. It's time to look at ourselves from a completely different perspective. Imagine you just arrived here, with no past or future. Now there is no story you are telling yourself. Remember, the future is always based upon a past, so in actuality, the future is the past. We are all time travelers in the realest sense. So simply imagine you just arrived here with no past or future. Simply remain in the now. How do we do that, you ask? Without effort, actually…

Imagine carrying around bags of groceries in both hands. Eventually your hands, arms, shoulders, neck, and back become strained. It's exhausting carrying around those groceries all the time. Imagine if I said to you, "Just put the groceries down. It's okay."

"Are you sure? I've been carrying these forever. I can really put them down?"

"Yes. Just put them down."

There is no effort or straining in putting them down, in letting go. All the effort and strain is in carrying them. Put your groceries of past and future down. Just gently place them on the floor. You will instantaneously feel lighter, freer, happier, and healthier. There is no need to pick them back up. You can if you want; they'll be there waiting for you, I promise. All your suffering will return the moment you pick them back up. Just leave them here with me. Now you can use your energy much more effectively and creatively without strain.

Psychologically speaking, a human being is just memory. You have memorized the meanings of all these words, so there is no need to "think" in order to understand or communicate via speech. You see a chair; you know how to use it. You see a cup; you know how to drink from it. You know how to drive your car, wash yourself, feed yourself, groom yourself. There is not a single aspect of your life that hasn't been memorized. There is no need to think about anything.

Eventually this new understanding of non-ego mind or a true meditative state will be your way of living. This is a far superior way of life. It's how we repair and self-heal our body of energy. It's how we can feel the joy, completeness, and happiness inherent within the Self. This new meditative state will allow you to feel energized and fulfilled because you needn't carry the groceries of your false identity all the time. These things are not you, and neither is all your disease and suffering.

By living this way, you're continually infusing your body of energy with the higher frequencies of the immortal Self. Remember, what is original to you is perfection, divinity, and completeness. There is no disharmony, disease, and dysfunction within your sentience, which is what we really are. This is how to truly live, as what is original to you. Now we can see how to be clear-minded and relaxed and still get things done. We do everything better, with more imagination, more power, and more joy, when we are the Self. Try it and see what happens.

Freedom from the known awakens the true limitless imagination of human potential.

Client Example: Prescription Drug Addiction, Pain, Depression, Anxiety

Barbara is a very talented graphic artist who has battled prescription drug addiction, pain, anxiety, and depression for over ten years. She attempted to get off drugs numerous times, only to relapse each and every time. With each relapse, she would hit a deeper and deeper level of depression, anxiety, and self-loathing. Her sister was worried that she might overdose. Barbara initially hurt her back skiing as an Olympic hopeful back in high school. The constant pain and dashed dreams eventually led to her depression, anxiety, and addiction to pain meds.

Barbara had been prescribed countless pharmaceuticals for many, many years and had earnestly tried several rehab facilities with absolutely no improvement or increase in her quality of life. She could not take her career as a graphic artist to the heights that were reflective of her talent, and was desperately running out of time with her battle with drug addiction.

I met Barbara through her younger sister, Tori, who attended a meditation class I was teaching. Tori was very concerned that her sister's self-destructive behavior would eventually take her past the point of no return. She felt that Barbara could not control her negative thoughts or say no to her cravings. Tori didn't know where to turn anymore and brought her to the next meditation class. I could feel both her desperation and her love for her sister, and I knew she felt Barbara was in a dangerous place in terms of her mental and physical health.

During the meditation class, Barbara briefly experienced for the first time a profound stillness and silence. It was so impactful that she immediately decided she wanted to work with me.

We got to the core of her suffering in our first session.

"I've been like this for years. It feels like my mind, emotions, and constant pain are out of my control, RJ."

"That's because all of your energy has become looped, repeatedly and addictively misdirected at the behest of your egoic identity's identifications. It's like cutting across your backyard along the exact same path every single time. Eventually the grass gets crushed and dies. The path just gets wider and more defined. This is what habits do to us. They pull more and more of our energy down the same well-trodden path, leaving us less and less empowered to change."

Barbara's eyes got wider. "That's exactly how I feel."

"Eventually this habitual disharmony became your normal way of being. This now-normalized disharmonious energy pattern literally reformats you, energetically. Belief, thought, emotion, action, and behavior literally reshape us. This disharmony is then represented in changes to our genes, DNA, proteins, and cells. This is part of why overcoming addiction or even physical injury can be so challenging. When the driving force in your life is a disempowering, disharmonious, nonaccepting, and non-loving perspective (your belief-based egoic identity), you take yourself out of balance and literally create your experience of discomfort, disease, and ill health. This vicious cycle of suffering spirals downward until the body of energy can no longer function properly and becomes damaged beyond repair."

"Wow, you just described my life. It makes me feel sick."

"It's okay," I said. "That's Barbara's life, and you're not Barbara. You simply created her. You have been living through her, with your attention upon her, for so long that you lost all perspective and completely forgot she isn't really you. You are perfect, complete, and free. Barbara isn't, and it's why she suffers and is sick."

Barbara's eyes watered: "The idea of separation fills me with such...emotion. I feel this space between who I really am and my persona. I want to really get this, though. It feels like trying to catch soap bubbles, grabbing on to this knowing."

"I understand. First, you want to keep working on that feeling and recognition of space you talked about. The more you get yourself there, the more you'll want to move into that space because it feels so good. And it feels so good because you are actually feeling your true essence—the Self—without your energy being manipulated by the egoic identity. The more you practice this, the easier it will get."

You can find the meditation I taught Barbara after this story. When we completed the practice, Barbara said, "That was incredible. I see how I do not create thoughts as part of my Real Self, but rather that they are something the egoic identity creates using energy in order to reinforce a sense of itself."

"Brilliant. It does all of this for a sense of existence and security. We do the same with bodily sensations. Through pleasure and pain, we reinforce the authenticity of the false self and misidentification with the physical body."

"I had no idea this is how it works and how I don't have to use my energy to constantly think or emotionally identify with bodily sensations like pain. I certainly don't have to believe in thoughts or sensations so much that they affect me deeply."

After a few weeks of meditation, Barbara found a lovely space between her thoughts, emotions, and bodily sensations and her self-awareness of them. Subsequently, her thoughts, emotions, and pain began to have less and less of an impact on her. She felt better and better.

"Now I get it. If we were really our thoughts, feelings, and bodily experiences, when they passed, we would pass too. For instance, if I'm angry at my boyfriend for something he said, and he apologizes, it's all cool again. The anger's gone, but I'm not—so I'm not the anger."

"Exactly, Barbara. We often say things like 'I am angry or sad or dumb' without even realizing that we are identifying through emotion with the words 'I am.'"

"Wow, we do. I never thought of it that way. We create thoughts, emotions, and experiences, and then believe they are us. Now that I have space, I feel free inside."

She became adept enough to quiet her agitated mind. Barbara employed this meditation technique even during waking, working, everyday life. Her anxiety and emotional swings quickly began to dissipate because there was not the initial torrent of negative thoughts to trigger them. Her ability to manage her pain sensations increased dramatically as well. After two weeks, Barbara felt more relaxed, happier, and more like herself than ever before.

"The crazy thing is I'm going into that space all the time now. I'll be waiting at a red light, and I'll just start breathing into the hollow. Before I get out of bed, right before I go to sleep, and here and there throughout my day, I'll take a pause and connect directly to my essence."

"Exactly! The more you do it consciously, the more you'll start to do it subconsciously. You'll find yourself looking for opportunities to practice. Pretty soon, you'll always be your True Self."

Her struggle with prescription medications was harder for her to see clearly. We spoke about how her egoic identity was wrapped up in identifying with addiction and the physical body. She had long associated herself with either the flawed genetics of the body, her physical injuries, or the habitual and addictive behavior of drug use, and therefore saw herself as a victim to them. When total misidentification is the case, we cannot separate the self from the experience itself. This makes the misidentification impossible to transcend. Her eyes lit up at this revelation.

"I have always felt uncomfortable saying 'I'm a drug addict' over and over again. It's like I was marrying myself to it. Now I know why it never felt right."

"Repetition can create and reinforce misidentification. But some people need to say it out loud to others in order for it to be real. That's because the egoic identity is built upon everything that is outside the Self, so it is greatly affected by others' perceptions of it. This can make some people finally take responsibility in order to address it."

"I always felt much worse and more hopeless whenever I would say it."

"You were just ready to work with yourself in a different manner."

Through this meditation that I taught Barbara, along with the "Who am I?" exercise from earlier in the chapter, Barbara was able to directly experience the Self as pure awareness that simply uses energy to create. All projections, cravings, expectations, ruminations, thoughts, emotions, and behaviors belong to the belief-based egoic identity and misidentification with the physical body, none of which is direct sentience. Barbara was able to experience craving as separate from the Self. By observing the craving, she realized it was nothing she needed to act upon, no matter how persistent the urge. She used the meditation I taught her to simply remove the craving from her energy field. She did the exact same thing with pain signals.

Through our work together, Barbara began to clearly see the ritualized mental patterns of shame, guilt, and self-abuse within her body of energy. These patterns are hard to reroute or erase unless one goes to the source of these patterns. The step 1 exercises go to the Source within you. The old habitual and addictive thought patterns began to dissipate. Eventually the old, worn-out pathways of the false self were no longer consuming her energy. Her past was finally cleansed, and with it went the self-destructive addictions. The habit of disharmonious thoughts, emotions, actions, and behaviors was gone.

Barbara says she feels like she repaired, healed, and freed herself. She has done exactly that. Because she no longer identifies the Self with the physical body, her old skiing injuries no longer seem a part of who she really is inside. Her pain and fear of pain miraculously lessened through simple non-reaction and non-identification with the physical body. With her new understanding of herself, Barbara weened herself off her previous dosages through strict doctor supervision. Now CBD is more than enough to take the edge off when there is a flare-up of pain.

Barbara has since left behind her former toxic pattern of self-judgment and no longer imagines worst-case scenarios for her future. She can now truly be herself without being tied to the past or the future, all of which were projections of the egoic identity. It is the past or the future that brings the false self back into formation via thought. Now is the unsullied canvas on which to create without limitation.

Barbara is currently drug-free going on three years. She no longer suffers from crushing depression or severe anxiety. Her severe back and knee pain is nearly nonexistent. Her attitude toward herself and life has been transformed, and she feels eternally spacious and optimistic about everything. Her career as a graphic artist has taken a profound turn for the better, and she finds it much, much easier to navigate her personal life.

Step 1 Core Exercises:
Meditations to Log In to Your True Essence
Part 1: Feeling Your True Essence through Observation

Sit down in a chair, with your back supported and straight. Plant your feet firmly on the ground and rest your arms on the uppermost parts of your thighs, with your palms open and facing up.

Imagine yourself completely hollow, like an empty balloon with absolutely no insides, just a faint outline of form. Breathe in, utilizing the diaphragm, and fill the empty space inside you with life force upon each inhale. As you exhale, imagine you are expelling every belief, bone, thought, emotion, and experience. Empty yourself, through your exhale, of all that you filled your container with. Repeat and repeat and repeat until you have emptied yourself of any accumulated history or projected future. Empty yourself until what remains is simply a hollow, perfect container that houses only pure beingness. The outline of your entire container is awareness held in place by the life force itself. Remember, what you really are is formless, free, and unconditioned.

Watch as your belief-based egoic identity becomes active. It's addicted to the movement of the past, which is thinking. Thinking is the only way the false self can exist. See and feel the energy moving up your hollow body into your mental body just above and outside your container. See the play of thought, because you are feeding the mental body with energy. See how the egoic mind has taken control, because it is a parasite, obsessed with itself. Just feel and watch the energy leaving its center point beneath your belly button and above the groin and going up and out of your hollow container into the mental body like a cartoon bubble.

Observe that if you run with a thought, and believe in it, you will automatically bathe it in an emotion. See how that brings the bubble of thought closer to your container, into the emotional body, as though it's pressing down on your container. Recognize where the emotion fueled by misidentification sits upon your container.

Now simply cease to believe in the emotion's authenticity. It has no actual vitality or staying power. It's all your creation, all your doing, and it's all empty. Just let it go. It's not you.

Inhale deeply, fill your hollow self with the energetic life force, and exhale the emotion and thought that were sitting atop your outline of form. See the emptiness in what you created. Tangibly see the power you have to let all your creations go just by using your breath and intention.

Part 2: Logging In to Assess Your Energy

Pretend you just arrived here, with no past and no future. Feel the presence of Self within the center of your chest. Stay there. Touch your fingers to the center of your chest. Bring all of your attention and focus to the sensation of touch in the center of your chest. Close your eyes. Gently reach out from inside your chest and touch your fingertips.

This will directly activate your sentience while simultaneously opening your heart chakra. Stay within this. Gently feel your inner awareness, your inner sight, opening from inside your chest. Stay there. Do not judge or analyze anything. As you effortlessly reside within your inner awareness, tangibly see what is within your body of energy. Locate and recognize where any imbalance exists through your heightened inner perception. This imbalance could be physical pain, emotional discomfort, or mental anguish. Simply recognize where it is located and what it feels like.

Once any imbalance has been located, ask yourself, "To whom has this imbalance arisen?" The answer will be "to me." Then ask yourself, "Who am I?" You will get no answer. Dwell in the no-mind—the meditative state—and simply let the imbalance float away—because it will—or remove it energetically with your intention just like you would wave your hand to dismiss something. Repeat as needed until there is cessation and cleansing of any and all imbalances. If discomfort still persists, use the fingers to chest, and upon reaching out from inside the chest to touch your fingers, see and feel your heart opening so wide that its power ejects and removes any and all energetic imbalances within your field of energy. Repeat as needed.

❄ ❄ ❄

When you are truly ready to move past what you have been holding on to, as well as projecting into the future, the healer (the Real You) will appear. Once we begin to access and work with the Self directly, you'll experience clarity, connectivity, peace, freedom, empowerment, and better health.

Once the Self has been experientially known, you can ask yourself the most important question you can ever pose: "What is it that I am trying to achieve?" This is the focus of the next step.

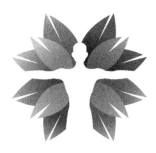

Step 2

Know Specifically What You Are Going to Achieve

My direct understanding is that the order of creation is desire, intention, thought, emotion, action, and then behavior. Nothing happens, so to speak, until there is desire. This is where we begin with step 2. Desire sets creation into motion, and when desire is attuned to God or the source of creation itself within, perfection is created. Once your desire is fully formalized and agreed upon, your intention to achieve your desire can be activated. Once this intention is fixed, it becomes your will. The will is the most powerful force we have as a creator being, and it is tangibly experienced while we are incarnate. Your will is then translated into a thoughtform. Once that thoughtform is bathed in emotion through identification with the thought, it becomes actionable. We did this in step 1. Now your larger body of energy has been fully activated by the electric current, or the energetic life force, you just harnessed within you. We then arrive at the "actions" we perform in order to make something come to fruition in physical reality.

The ultimate state of self-awareness is to be consciously aware of the motivation behind your every desire, intention, thought, emotion, action, and behavior. This clarity is power itself and renders all obstacles and opponents powerless. This is Self-Mastery and is the subject matter I will teach and deconstruct in upcoming books.

Energetically, the first component of creation—desire—exists within a much higher frequency compared to the other components of creation. With each subsequent component, we drop like a Slinky going down the steps in frequency. This means pure desire exists in a higher-vibrational environment or state, followed by intention, and then thought, emotion, action, and finally behavior. Often without consciously realizing it, we fine-tune our desire until it becomes specific. Once the specificity is determined, we use our intention by harnessing our energy into lower-frequency thought about how to do it. Once the thoughts are bathed in an emotion through identification, which is an even lower frequential realm than thought, they are now actionable and are brought forth into the physically perceivable realms, which consist of the lowest possible frequencies. The physical body now has been sufficiently electrically charged into action in order to satiate the desire. Metaphysically speaking, this is how we operate when human.

You are the most powerful when operating at the higher frequencies of desire and intention. Once you have dropped frequency into the lower realms of thought, emotion, action, and behavior, the purity, efficacy, and power of your energy has been diminished. It (your original desire) has also become highly susceptible to the influence of your egoic identity and all low-frequency stimuli. Working directly with the Self negates the issue of weakened efficacy and purity inherent within the lower frequencies. Namely, it keeps you energetically operating above the corruption of your egoic identity and the low frequency of your local physical environment. Picture how oil rests atop the water while contained within the same glass.

When I was told that I was permanently paralyzed from the chest down, I had one very specific desire: to walk again. I knew this accomplishment, this healing, was contained within me. I would simply bring this knowingness and healing into my experiential reality. Bringing about my desired result required a total union of my specific desire, unwavering will, and complete detachment. I knew this would take every ounce of my life force: in other words, I had to perpetually maintain a clear, specific, and unwavering single-pointedness of focus without tension. However long and whatever physical, emotional, and mental toll this accomplishment would exact was of absolutely no consequence. This is the mindset of victory.

Once we know what we want to achieve, we must marry ourselves to this goal. Achievement, reality, and Total Self become one. There can be no doubt, which means no egoic mind and all its limiting chatter getting in the way of our desired result. We must fix our intent, unequivocally and unbroken, on this desired result while simultaneously not reaching for it. Once we do, the achievement that is already contained within can become tangibly known. It's no different than the powerful tree that already exists within the tiny seed. That specific internal state of being just needs to be brought into tangible manifestation. To do this, we must harness the Total Self (sentience + complement of energy) powerfully. This is not a mere mental understanding or emotional connection. What I am talking about exists prior to that and is a vibration deep within the Self. Once we marry and meld our will to the fulfilled achievement that already exists within us, its manifestation into our physical reality is inevitable.

Our unwavering, fixed, permanent intention is our will, and it is the power of creation itself.

The Power of Intention

Intention and the subsequent Slinky drop-down in frequency to the realms of thought, emotion, action, and behavior truly shape and co-create our inner and outer worlds. Everything happens because of our intention, period. The life you created is a result of your intentions. There is nothing that manifests in our outer world that did not have its genesis of desire and intention from within. Once you harness the Self properly, including the higher frequencies of your desire and intention, you become a master creator instead of a master of limitations.

Your doubt (low frequency) is what throws water on the fire of your intention (high frequency). Doubt is death and is a product of your false created self. When you look at doubt and its source, it is always the finite mind. Doubt is simply the low-frequency misuse of your imagination.

When we work at the desire/intention level, we bring the higher realms of consciousness into the lower realm of physical reality. This is operating above the lower frequencies of thought, emotion, and physicality. Instead, we are *creating* at the higher frequencies of pure desire and intention. Remember that the order of creation is desire, intention, thought, emotion, action, and then behavior. These vibrations are also descendent in terms of frequency, with desire being the highest vibration of creation and behavior being the lowest.

When we work with pure desire and a fixed intention, we utilize a higher, more powerful, and more effective vibrational force in which the lower frequencies are directly and potently influenced. When you do this, you operate closer to the source of Self. Both this higher frequency and its manifestation are already contained within you. You're simply bringing this achievement "out" into the lower frequencies where it can be physically perceived.

The more specific you are about what you desire to achieve, the more you fine-tune your ability as a creator. This powerfully unleashes your full intention to manifest your desire into experiential reality.

Once you clear your awareness of all imaginary limitations from step 1, which are your past ruminations and future projections, then you can objectively and specifically see your desired end result. If you are no longer bound by imaginary ruminations or expectations, you are now ready to create powerfully. This allows you a new understanding, and the openness to intuitively know what you need to work with and upon in order to achieve your desired result. What is needed from moment to moment in order for your achievement to manifest into experiential reality is the single-pointedness of true clarity and your limitless power that authentic freedom engenders.

Addressing Doubt

Keep in mind that doubt is limitation itself. It throws water on the fire of your intention. Remove all doubt. Its source is always the incomplete false self. Both the false self and doubt are transient and limited. Imagination and the Total Self are not. Only doubt can stop the electronic force of your will. Doubt is a contradictory electrical impulse that stops the flow of your intention and sends an alternate electrical impulse toward a different result.

For example, Bob wants to close a sale on a mansion. He focuses on the contract being signed by all parties, issuance of the new deed, and his commission check. But his last five sales have fallen through, so his egoic mind is trying to prepare him for failure in order to protect him. This contradictory intention (preparing for the deal to fall through) interferes with his desired intention (the sale going through and his earning a big commission). Without his entire intention focused on the sale, he loses the power of manifesting it. Even worse, when another sale starts to brew, his egoic mind will remind him not only of his previous six fails but also that "doing all of that silly intending didn't work."

I'm as serious as a sheet of flame when I say doubt is the death of intention. Stay away from it, always. Doubt, my friends, literally creates an alternative reality to your original intention. If doubt pops in, simply ask yourself, "Who is it that doubts?" Answer: "Me. I am the one who doubts." Ask yourself, "Who am I?" You will get no answer and the doubt will cease to have any negative power over your consciousness and energy.

When we are first inspired to achieve a specific goal, the egoic identity may still be quite active, so what we desire to achieve may seem impossible to our program of limitations. In fact, well-meaning, educated, and compassionate people may offer their experiences, beliefs, and knowledge (all past limitations that have nothing to do with you) regarding what's possible and what's not. For me, while I appreciated and respected my neurosurgeon, infectious disease doctor, endocrinologist, primary care MD, nurses, aides, and physical therapists, I never took a single word they said onboard. And the same was true for the input I received from all the other paraplegics and quadriplegics. By never identifying with any of these perceived stimuli, I was unencumbered by any external limitations. My will never wavered. Not. Even. Once.

There cannot be a single thought or feeling of doubt that the desired result will not be realized. If your glorious intention is a raging inferno, doubt is a bucket of water that douses your flame. If you say to yourself, "I need to get up and go to work," your physical body will follow that electrical impulse and begin doing what needs to be done in order to get you to work. In order for that current of energy to be disrupted, you must send a contradictory electrical impulse to stop that current flow of electricity. When you then say, "Nah, I don't feel like going to work today," you stop the original direction of electricity and send an alternate current. The physical body will then respond to that new directive and an alternate reality is now created. You may suddenly feel tired, unsettled, or even ill because the mind has supplied a reason for staying home.

Bottom line: All the promises you make to yourself that you do not keep are little defeats to your will. Eventually the totality of your capitulations makes you feel defeated before you even try to achieve your next goal. Do not break your will, ever, under any circumstances. Once there is no separation between your will and you, you are *invincible*. You have become one with what you will achieve. How long it takes to manifest or how it happens is of absolutely no consequence, except to the limited false self. Just know the transformation process is underway, and you are simply utilizing your will to manifest this achievement that is already within you. It is no different from when you type a destination into your GPS. You know you are going to get there, and because you know this, you never doubt it. You simply focus on what you need to do from moment to moment. Know that your healing already resides within the deepest levels of your existence, because it does. Once the will begins to manifest, what was once impossible to the egoic mind becomes inevitable for the Self.

In my case, in order to maintain the single-pointedness of my intention, I removed all contact with family and friends because I refused to leak any of my energetic power by explaining what had happened, the diagnosis, how I felt, what antibiotics I was taking, what type of surgery I'd had, when I would be discharged, and all the other questions that well-meaning people ask. This explaining and rehashing was a waste of my energy because it did not serve what I was trying to achieve: the transcendence of permanent paralysis and severe disease. I knew that nothing could stop me from walking again except a lack of my fully harnessed indomitable will and the complete detachment from any result. It is being able to simultaneously hold the paradox of the iron will and complete detachment and non-identification with any future result that unleashes your power to transform. Perpetually and potently stay in the realm of transcendent creativity. Never forget this, my friends.

Step 2 Shortcuts to Separate Yourself from Your Doubts

Here are some practices you can make use of to help counter any doubts you may have.

Countering Doubt Pop-Ins

In step 1's shortcut practices in the previous chapter, there were two that you should refer back to in order to counter doubts that pop into your mind. These practices are "Clear Old Disharmonious Thought Patterns" and "Clear Old Disharmonious Emotional Patterns" on pages 71–72.

Unfollow Your Doubts

One way to help separate yourself from doubt is to unfollow or mute those you follow on social media or step away from it entirely for a while. You can craft a note of explanation to give to friends and family, letting them know about certain topics you don't want to discuss while you are in your healing mode. You could also designate someone else to do this for you if you don't want to focus your energy on it.

Here is a sample letter that you can build on when creating your own letter.

Dear (blank),

As you may or may not know, I have been tasked with a personal health challenge that requires my complete attention and full focus. Moving forward, I will be refraining from my usual interactions and communications in order to harness my energies in the needed direction for the return of my health and greater well-being. This is not a personal slight, judgment, or rebuke of you or anyone in any way. I have simply chosen to be single-minded in my focus in order to give myself the energy and attention I need to heal at this time. If you wish to receive updates about me or have questions, please contact (blank). I thank you in advance for your respect and understanding regarding my decision to focus on myself at this time.

❋ ❋ ❋

In addition to the permanent chest-down paralysis, I was also diagnosed with sepsis, type 1 diabetes, hypothyroidism, Hashimoto's disease, pancreatitis, a retracted heart, and a nodular thyroid. I was physically weak beyond belief. So I would not and could not waste a single breath, thought, emotion, or action. Every bit of energy and intention needed to be directly in line with what I was going to achieve through the fixed intention of my indomitable will and the complete detachment from any future result. I maintained a permanent state of powerful conscious creation. I asked Jennifer to tell everyone to please not contact me. She would provide updates to them. I never gave this situation another thought, and Jennifer never again mentioned well-meaning family members and friends who wanted to talk to me. They respected my wishes, and the people closest to me, upon hearing of the severity of my hopeless situation, even told Jennifer they expected me to fully recover.

The healing opportunity and space I created and accessed *within* myself extended outward as well. I did not have any disturbances while in the rehabilitation hospital. I requested that my door be shut at all times. I refused to *accept* any noise, conversation, or negative energy from the hallway that would affect my process of manifesting my healing. My only recurring guest was my acupuncturist, Adrian. Jennifer was unable to visit me due to her own severe back injury that would eventually require surgery. She kept the severity of her injury from me during our daily video chats, as she literally could not sit or walk.

My hospital room was a high-frequency zone because of my elevated state of consciousness. It was so peaceful that staff members would ask if they could silently sit in my room while they were on their lunch break. The high-frequency healing energy was palpable.

Think about people you've been around who leave you out of sorts, depressed, or drained. Or those who lift your frequency and make you feel peaceful, joyful, and uplifted. That's proof of how our own frequency affects others—and how theirs affects us. You must always be aware of your frequency and that of the environment around you. It's for your own protection to stay away from those who affect you adversely during your healing process.

Let nothing interfere with what you're trying to achieve. Everything must be in accordance with the single-pointedness of precisely what you want to achieve. If something isn't, remove it immediately. Remove all obstacles, both physical and intangible. I had all the literature and videos regarding how to live with paralysis as well as disease removed from my hospital room. I replaced them with a gentle mister for aromatherapy and crystals. I kindly but forcibly told the staff that I had no interest in hearing stories of all those patients who came before me who did not recover from their traumatic spinal injury and severe chronic illness. Instead, I offered to explain one time how I would heal myself of chest-down paralysis and severe illness. That, on occasion depending upon my energy level, I would briefly elaborate on if they wished to sincerely discuss it with me. If there are no more obstacles, no more limitations, and your unwavering intention is permanently fixed and fully unionized with the Total Self, there exists nothing but the inevitable manifestation of the achievement.

I never had a single thought that I wouldn't walk again. Not one. A true Master Creator only thinks about what it intends to manifest. The transient egoic identity is limitation itself, and mine had been destroyed along with my physical body. My old operating system had been eradicated. It was replaced with an enhanced, more powerful, and sensitive processor: cosmic consciousness. I was in a state of grace and was totally free even though my body had been destroyed and I couldn't feel or move from the chest down. I had awakened.

My physical body was so damaged that I couldn't even cough or gather enough air in my lungs to laugh. To move my legs a fraction of an inch was an impossibility. I saw healing my body as a challenge, nothing more, nothing less. I gave this challenge absolutely no weight. I simply accepted that the body was experiencing temporary paralysis and that the temporary placeholder, the fictional character called RJ, had been diagnosed with the infection and all the diseases. That's how I verbalize it. I never identified with any of it, and therefore it didn't have any power over me. Never. I accepted it as something to simply work with and transcend. And so it shall be for you!

Don't be fooled by your expectations. They're also a form of limitation. Unless what you're trying to achieve comes in your expected form or anticipated route, you will not be open to the infinite possibilities the achievement can manifest, and therefore it will not be in your realm of perception. In this sense, expectations even of the grandest sense are actual limitations. The finite mind cannot see this, but the luminous eyes of timeless wisdom are never blinded.

Client Example

Carl is in his mid-thirties and a well-known entrepreneur. He, his accomplished wife, and their five young children live in New York City and have for many years. When he was referred to me, he was suffering from high stress, which had led to a large weight gain and subsequent health issues. His self-image, due to the weight gain, had developed into a crushing fear of public speaking, all of which were negatively impacting his career and personal life.

During our first video remote session, Carl shared that he leads his entire company's innovation, which relies on his genius-level, creative problem-solving abilities. He was expected to exceed expectations for his internationally renowned corporate clients and meet one tight deadline after another. His battle with stress and subsequent health challenges created doubt in his ability to keep outdoing himself. In addition to his own responsibilities, he had to make sure his company was performing at the highest levels possible.

I explained step 2 to him, of knowing exactly what you are going to achieve through desire and setting intention, and asked what he wanted to achieve during our time together. He said he wanted to achieve four very specific things: alleviate his stress, lose weight and get healthy, feel confident that his creativity would not run dry, and overcome his now acute fear of public speaking.

First, I addressed how true creativity never wanes, because it's the activity of the higher mind. This entire book and how I help others is from a similar perspective. Higher consciousness accesses the information beyond the low frequencies. It's the low frequencies that create the finite mind. Carl is a creative genius and is able to consistently outdo himself because he's able to stay consistently attuned to his higher mind. I explained that everything already exists, and truly creative people like Carl are simply tapping into what is beyond the realm of our five physical senses and intellect. This revelation greatly eased Carl's doubt regarding his ability to perpetually deliver on a high level. He reported that within one week, his stress level markedly dissipated and his self-confidence at delivering at genius-level creativity returned.

Next, we tackled Carl's weight gain and subsequent poor health. Carl was specific and stated that he wanted to lose thirty pounds and lower his blood sugar by one-third. I instructed him to begin eating just two meals a day (always at the same times and intervals) that combined would not exceed twelve hundred calories. He must avoid all processed foods and starchy carbohydrates and limit dairy. His body needed vegetables, nuts, and lean proteins in order to slim down, have energy, and reduce insulin levels. (In the appendix of this book, I go into great detail, from a higher consciousness perspective, regarding diet and fasting, what really happens, and when repair/healing occurs within the body.) I also told Carl he could enjoy as much green tea and black coffee as desired for mental acumen and digestion. Within two weeks of implementing these changes, Carl lost ten pounds and his daily blood sugar readings had dropped twenty-five percent. He could not believe how much better he felt on multiple levels.

His final desire, to overcome his recent but overwhelming fear of public speaking, was a bit more nuanced. "I had to cancel my last two presentations with huge international corporations because the thought of presenting in front of the board of directors was too much for me."

"Too much for who?"

"For me. I feel like I am going to screw it up as soon as I open my mouth."

"Who feels like they are going to screw it up?"

"I do. I can feel that they are judging me about my weight. I get too nervous now and I know I'll just lose the account."

This was a big admission for Carl. Now that he was totally honest, we could specifically address the problem from a different perspective.

"Carl, none of that is true. Your egoic identity is the false who that thinks and feels this way. You are simply identifying with passing phenomena, like thoughts and feelings."

The beginnings of a smile began to curl around the corners of Carl's mouth as he recognized the truth of what was just said.

"I felt that. That makes sense. But how do I stop doing this? Because once it starts, it snowballs fast."

"When you are doing a presentation, what are you trying to achieve?"

"To close the sale."

"No, that's an ancillary effect of a powerful presentation. What is the original primary objective you are trying to achieve by giving the presentation?"

Carl lowered his gaze from mine as he searched within himself for the answer. Then it hit him.

"To clearly present the elegance and power of my solution to their problem in an engaging way."

"Exactly. All of your creative genius and formidable acumen will be fine-tuned and online by fully engaging yourself in exactly what you are trying to achieve. Then there is no opportunity for any contradictory thoughts or feelings to occur."

Those earlier tiny beginnings of a smile now spread wide across his face. I could see and feel the weight of self-doubt being lifted.

"I can't believe it's that simple. All that stress and anxiety. I totally forgot the whole point of my presentations and why I used to love doing them."

"Now that you consciously know what you are specifically trying to achieve during your presentations, you can fully immerse yourself in that once again. You will automatically be supremely engaged. At that deep level of Total Self-activation, the egoic mind and all its self-judgment disappears. And with it, so will your fears about public speaking."

That week, Carl rescheduled his previous two presentations. Two weeks later, he closed an eight-figure deal after blowing away the board of directors. Over the next four months, Carl lost a grand total of forty pounds and has successfully returned to better health, including an over thirty percent drop in his blood sugar levels. Mission accomplished.

Step 2 Core Exercise: Set Your Intention and Desire

Perform the following exercise only once, and the egoic identity's fears will no longer consume your energy. First, repeat the step 1 exercise "Feeling Your True Essence through Observation" on pages 82–83 until you are completely calm, totally clear, and fully present. Then move on to this portion of practice for step 2:

- Breathe deeply from the diaphragm. This aligns your conscious mind directly with your sentience.
- Follow the breath, not your thoughts, until the mind and body are calm.
- Then, and only then, ask yourself this question: "What is it that I am trying to achieve?"
- Let the sentience deep within answer the question.
- Write down your answer. Do not analyze it or correct the first response. This is your initial desire. Look at it deeply.
- Read the words that you've written out loud and feel the meaning of each word.
- See if this statement needs further clarification or could be more specific. If so, repeat steps 1 and 2. Ask yourself, "Is this exactly what I am trying to achieve?"
- Modify the initial desire and write it down.
- Look at it again deeply.
- Feel the meaning of every word and see if it deeply and perfectly resonates.
- Ask yourself once more, "Is this precisely what I am trying to achieve?"

- Make the adjustment from your modified desire to your final desire and write it down one last time.
- Stare at the words you've written.
- Is this statement the truest, most specific and accurate desire that you want to achieve? If not, modify it again through the process outlined in the bullet points.
- When you have uncovered precisely, and without a shadow of a doubt, what you're trying to achieve, write it down one last time, clearly, with the finality of complete conviction.

❋ ❋ ❋

What started as a mere question has now been transformed into your specific and fixed intention. The future steps of the ATFHT will bring this intention into tangible reality.

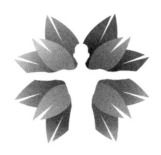

Step 3
Activate Your Healing Intention

Step 3 is about activating the state of healing with the intention you created in step 2. This step can be thought of in this way: mental visualization + physical action + emotional stimulation + the spoken word = full activation of your healing intention. When we combine mental visualization, physical movement, emotional stimulation, and the spoken word concurrently, we have brought together the four rudimentary expressions of the human form to supercharge our single-pointedness of healing.

Early on while I performed rehabilitation exercises, or, more accurately, had physical therapists manipulate my body because I couldn't on my own, I appeared to be completely zoned out. A more accurate description is that I was totally tuned in. I visualized myself already having performed the exercise perfectly. I remembered, within my every fiber and cell, what it felt like to have sensation and functionality within my body. I tangibly knew what sensation felt like and that perfection was always contained within me. I verbally expressed my intention while I exercised or while being manually manipulated with the command "I am the conqueror of my mind and body." I also repeated that invocation constantly, utilizing the mentally spoken word. I didn't just say these words; I saw, meant, and felt them with complete and total conviction.

A command directed by your sentience powerfully summons your body of energy. While you rehabilitate your health or injury, incorporate all of the rudimentary human expressions to transform your body of energy. Harness your preferred avenue of consciousness, as we discussed in the previous chapter, into a single-pointedness of intention. Harness it completely, utterly, and unleash the power of transformation through your will. Recognize the improved energy flow and bring it into experiential reality to heal yourself.

Once you master this step, it will be a ninja-level form of rejuvenation for your body of energy. You, and only you, are the sentience and power to command yourself in totality. Only you, and you alone, for all eternity. *Now* is the time to reclaim this mastery.

Through your verbal command, your favored avenue of consciousness, physical movement, visualized perfect execution, and tangible remembrance, you make it so. Through your practice of this step, you will feel the revitalizing life force flow through your damaged areas as your activated state commands it. You are repairing and rebuilding yourself.

This step harmonizes the totality of the lower consciousness. Along with the other steps, it unleashes transformation. My healing was incredibly rapid and miraculous, beyond what healthcare professionals had any frame of reference for. I employed these four aspects (visualizing, physical action, emotional connection, and the spoken word) as much as possible.

Do not waste a single opportunity to employ every available resource to facilitate and manifest healing. Even while I was in my hospital bed, when one of the physical therapists would stretch my legs before and after my rehab session, I would employ this step. In my mind's eye, I would see me walking as before paralysis, tangibly remember what walking felt like, emotionally connect with that feeling deep inside my physicality, and then command the experience into now by verbalizing it. We can make the cells, proteins, neurons, tissue, and muscles repair themselves. They are simply energy. We can command it! All energy takes orders from the more sentient and powerful force—the Real You. You'll learn how to do this in the core exercise for step 3 at the end of this chapter.

Our direct, unwavering, focused intention is the power of creation itself.

If the thought of verbalizing your intention in front of people seems like it could be embarrassing, ask yourself, "Who is it that's worried about feeling embarrassed?" *Me, I am.* "Who am I?" The egoic identity's program of limitations is the root cause of disease and disharmony. Silence the belief-based egoic mind and never look back. Never.

When I spoke aloud my intentions, my therapists would immediately encourage me. They became even more inspired for me to stand and walk again. I could feel their added excitement and intention aid in my healing. I could utilize their energy just like when you get a pep talk. I could feel them being inspired by me, and I was by them. It was beautiful, transcendent—and powerful.

Bathing your intention with the life force of breath through the use of speech, along with the above mental/emotional/physical components, fully activates and incorporates the rudimentary creative expressions of humanity. You are "spelling" your body of energy to repair and self-heal. Have no doubt about this—and have no doubt that Merlin the Great would be proud of you!

Client Example: Dance Injuries, Debilitating Pain, Opioid Dependency

An emotionally intelligent special education teacher in her early thirties, Rebecca had been an exceptional athlete since childhood. But her constant pain from ankle injuries and surgeries, and her inability to continue her active and rugged lifestyle, led to an opioid dependency that she had suffered through for three years before I met her. Her high-energy, positive outlook on life had been replaced by depression, frustration, and chronic pain.

I met with Rebecca in person at my office, and at first glance, the effects of her physical and mental confusion were obvious. She did not walk freely, nor was she free mentally or emotionally. Bound by the energetic thievery of the belief-based egoic identity, she exuded an unhappiness, along with a constant preoccupation with the sensations of physical discomfort. I could also recognize a fairly advanced level of sentience straining to get out of her ritualized, self-imposed prison of identifications.

I asked her to sit down. "What is it that you would like to achieve through us working together?"

She said, "My friend Candace told me you've healed people from all sorts of injuries. I have some severe ones I want fixed."

I nodded. "I can sense damage to your knees and ankles and a recent injury to your right hip. Is that accurate?"

She smiled. I'd passed her test. "You got it. I hurt my hip two days ago. My ankles and knees have been damaged for years. I've been taking pain medications since 2014. I just don't feel like myself anymore." She pressed her lips together but couldn't stop them from quivering. "I can't work out or be physically active like I used to. It's my passion. I just want to be able to feel that joy again." Then she let the torrent come, one she'd obviously been holding back all of those years. She cried so hard that her shoulders were shaking and she had a hard time talking.

I said nothing. I simply held a high frequency so she could unburden herself. I do this by keeping my conscious focus above the lower realms of thought, emotion, and physicality.

Finally she regained control, tossing her wadded-up tissue in the trash can. "I want *me* back. I don't like the person I've become. I have no purpose. I'm depressed, in pain, and angry."

"Who are you angry with?"

"Me," she said without hesitation. "I don't like me."

I was so glad she'd worded it that way. Rebecca admitting this to herself was the open door. Now we could get to work.

I smiled at her, which she responded to with a puzzled look. "Rebecca, you are a beautiful soul. I wish you could see what I see. If you did, all of this nonsense would stop immediately."

Now she frowned, crossing her arms in front of her chest defensively. "What nonsense?"

The egoic identity, the source of all suffering, defends itself, as it always does, in order to have dominion over the divinity, freedom, and perfection of the Self.

I said, "Everything you just said is total nonsense. Not a single word has a shred of truth to it. I cannot help anyone who doesn't truly want to help themselves."

She opened her mouth to speak, and closed it again. She was coming to terms with the realization that I wasn't going to do all the work to heal her. It just doesn't work that way.

"Rebecca, stop thinking and look at me."

She glanced at me and quickly looked away again.

"Really look into my eyes," I said. "What do you *see*?"

She stared deeply, sincerely trying to connect. "Kindness." Her eyes widened as she went to the next level. "A cosmic intelligence. A higher power."

"That's *you*, Rebecca. You can perceive only what is already within you. *You* are those things. I am just the mirror."

Something shifted for her in that moment. The truth was registering. I could feel the dissipation of fog that thoughts and emotions create. "Hold my gaze, Rebecca. Keep connecting with what's behind my eyes."

As she did, she began to smile.

I said, "Now you see how everything you said earlier was total nonsense."

"Incredible. What did you do?"

"Nothing. You just reconnected with your Self. I didn't do a thing."

She laughed. "Really? I feel amazing. It didn't seem like I did anything."

"It took absolutely no effort on your part because this state is what you already and always are. Stop trying to convince yourself otherwise. Now, is this the 'me' that you missed?"

"Yes!"

"Okay, great. Are you ready to learn how to activate and direct your own repair and self-healing for your knees and ankles?"

"Of course," she said. "Why would you even ask that?"

"Because some people love their misery too much to let it go. They've misidentified themselves with their illness or injury for so long that sometimes their attachment to their symptoms and pain is their longest-standing relationship."

I could sense that statement really hit home. Rebecca unconsciously leaned back and clenched her fists.

"Are you willing to let go of all the things that cause your suffering?" I said. "It's the only way we heal ourselves."

She nodded, her face bright. "I'm willing."

"I am as well. Let's begin with the activated state."

I asked Rebecca to demonstrate the exercises her therapists taught her to rehabilitate her knees.

After she showed me the first exercise, I asked her to stop. "First, see yourself already performing the exercise perfectly. See it clearly in your mind's eye. Visualize the movement with as much detail as possible. Concentrate. Now tangibly remember what it feels like to move your legs that way. Don't reach out for the feeling. Instead, sink in and immerse yourself in it because the feeling is *within* you. Feel it deeply and totally. Swim in it. Now, as you're doing this, command your vital energy through the breath of life by saying, 'I repair and heal my knee now. With every movement, my knee is energized, repaired, and made strong.' Say these words with the sincerest devotion possible. Say them out loud. This is your command. Let the feeling well up from within your heart until you must verbalize it. Do not let the feeling pass, but rather give it expression through speech."

Rebecca did this but held back on the sincerity and devotion.

I leaned in. "Listen to me. You are far more powerful than that. Affect the energy that is your knee with the power that is your life force. Don't be shy. It's not befitting of such a perfect being."

The resonance in Rebecca's voice changed. I could feel the vibration rise and increase in power. Now we were getting somewhere.

"Now," I said, "perform your exercise as you perfectly imagined and felt it. Verbalize your command with sincerity and devotion. Do it now."

As Rebecca lifted her knee up to her chest and extended it fully outward, she stated, "I repair and heal my knee now. With every movement, my knee is energized, repaired, and made strong." She did it again. And again. And again. And again. She finally stopped. She smiled and opened her eyes. "My knee isn't clicking and it's not grinding like it normally does. It feels looser and cleaner inside. How is this possible?"

"Magick," I said. "Real magick."

After three weeks of constant healing activation via step 3, Rebecca told me that walking no longer caused pain. Her knees and ankles felt much better. She felt like she was commanding her repair and self-healing—and she was. Who else could be doing it? Two months later, she showed up at my office and flawlessly performed a little dance. Bravo, Rebecca!

Step 3 Core Exercise: Mental Visualization, Physical Action, Emotional Stimulation, and Spoken Word

In this practice you'll go through the steps of mentally visualizing, physically acting, stimulating your emotions/cellular memory, and verbalizing your command with sincerity and devotion in order to activate your healing state.

Mental Visualization

Close your eyes and picture yourself performing an activity that triggers your memory of past health, vitality, and joy. See it clearly in your mind's eye. Include as much detail as possible. Fixate completely on this image and this image only. Make this mental image your complete reality.

Physical Action

If you can keep your eyes closed while maintaining that mental image, perform, as much as you can, the very physical action. If you are unable to perform the full action, do a safer, limited version of it that simulates the recreated action. If need be, you can scale the action down to a safe and repeatable movement that precisely symbolizes the image you have in your mind's eye. Make the movement fully represent the image you have visualized. If you have a willing partner, have them assist you in your movement as needed.

Emotional Stimulation

While mentally seeing and physically performing your movement, remember, deep within your every fiber, what it felt like to perform that action. Feel it within every cell, muscle, and nerve. Lose yourself in that feeling once more as you see it in your mind's eye and are physically performing your action. Do not reach out for the feeling, but rather go deeply within and remember. Reignite your cellular, neurological, and muscle memory by bringing back that feeling fully and completely into now.

Spoken Word

Whatever your specific injury, ailment, or sickness entails, bring the remaining aspect of your life force into tangible, conscious fruition by verbalizing the following: "I repair and heal my (blank) now. With every movement, my (blank) is energized, repaired, and made whole once again." As much as you can, incorporate all four aspects simultaneously and in complete union. This will exponentially increase the efficacy of your fully activated healing state."

❄ ❄ ❄

By bringing the four aspects of self-expression into total cohesion, your highest potential or full amplification for self-healing is now activated. It is your certainty and completeness of this step (all the steps) that creates a higher-vibrational wave of powerful energy that courses through and completely permeates your entire being like nothing else can.

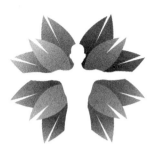

Step 4

Command Creator Consciousness

The building blocks of our physical form, which have been called energetic templates, originate and exist in much higher and significantly more subtle frequencies than our five physical senses perceive. By applying step 4, we learn how to access these higher states of consciousness and repair and heal ourselves at the root and not just treat symptoms. The tangible and direct experience of higher states of consciousness provides you with a greater sense of the expanded Total Self and subsequently an enhanced quality of life.

By now, you know that you're not the physical body (that's just the vehicle) or the egoic identity (that's the belief-based character we create). Through nonidentification with the finite mind's self-created program of limitations and nonidentification with the physical body, you can directly experience more of your Total Self and higher consciousness. Once your sentience has deepened and accrued sufficiently through experience, authentic self-realization becomes possible. It is from these exalted states of being that I tangibly understood how to heal my paralyzed and ravaged body. You, too, will eventually do this. Some of you are ready right now, and that is why this bolt of lightning is in your hands.

Step 4 provides access to the higher frequencies and dimensional constructs within and beyond the physical universe. The finite mind and its limited concepts of itself cannot function in states of limitless consciousness. You are going to discover higher frequencies where the energetic force of intention can co-create its reality instantaneously because of the faster, more holistic vibratory rate of the environment. This is a more expansive state of Creator Consciousness. In ancient texts, it was referred to as the realm of the gods.

Higher Intuitive Functions

The more sentient the entity/being is, the greater its bandwidth and sensitivity. Think of an old black-and-white TV set with the rabbit ears. Those antiquated devices have very limited bandwidth and poor receptivity. Now imagine today's smart TVs with super processors that provide incredible sensitivity, capabilities, and amazing functionality. More evolved sentience, when we access it directly, allows greater receptivity to its own wisdom, love, and power as well as these corresponding attributes within the Greater Reality. The deeper the reservoir of timeless wisdom and unconditional love, the more powerful and gentle you become. You realize the subtle and divine nature of existence while accessing the subtle and divine nature within yourself. This requires a different kind of inner attention and sensitivity.

This delicate and subtle yet powerful and illuminating inner awareness is represented by our higher intuitive functions, which, when seen as a whole, represent true Creator Consciousness. Higher intuitive functions can include, but are not limited to, the following:

- Clairsentience (intuitive knowing by feeling)
- Clairvoyance (intuitive knowing by seeing)
- Clairaudience (intuitive hearing)
- Claircognizance (intuitive knowledge, or wisdom)
- Clairempathy (intuitive feeling by emotion)
- Clairtaction (intuitive touch)
- Claireloquence (intuitive communicating)
- Clairolfactence (intuitive smell)

- Clairgustence (intuitive taste)
- Clairessence (intuitive embodiment, or the master of all intuitiveness)

These are not by any stretch of the imagination the totality of higher intuitive functions, but rather a small sampling of what you are capable of when you go beyond the very limited low-frequency realm of the physical senses, which produces our grandest delusion: so-called knowledge. You can think of sentience—the Self—as one gigantic eyeball—pure perception that has literally millions of sensors. Built into this screen of consciousness is your depth of self-understanding.

The ability to use your higher intuitive functions comes online as you surrender to the Self. They already exist within you. They are you, really. The combination of surrender and silence is kryptonite to the egoic identity and unleashes the true love, wisdom, and power of the Total Self.

When we are not using the more subtle and divine nature of attention, things are mistakenly labeled with a broad brush, such as judging something as simply conscious or not conscious. This misses the entire spectrum and degree of sentient self-awareness contained within the object being perceived. It's like judging a book by its cover or looking at a dolphin and assuming it's just a fish.

Recognizing Sentience

In regard to self-awareness and self-healing, understanding the difference between what you really are—sentience—and what you use to create—energy—is paramount. It is your sentient-directed energy that you will learn to use powerfully and properly in order to help heal the physical body. To easily and tangibly understand the difference between sentience and energy, all we have to do is examine ourselves. When you want to touch your head, it's your sentience that commands the energy within your body to lift your arm. This process of your sentience commanding the energy within your physical body to perform an act is constant and perpetual throughout your entire life. Your sentience commands the energy within your body, and within your larger body of energy. The body experiences your command as an electrical impulse through your nervous system that contracts the muscles in your arm, around your bones, in order to raise your hand to your head. Sentience commands our entire body of energy, always.

Thinking works the exact same way. Sentience commands energy into the mental body, which then uses the programs of logic and linearity to "think." We—sentience—simply have not achieved the prerequisite level of detachment with creations, such as belief, thought, emotions, or even the physical body, in order to master and heal our entire body of energy. Our primary and most intimate creation is the egoic identity, and we have become intoxicated by its delusions because we never take our attention off it. We lose the Self in our obsession with the egoic identity and, in the process, our freedom, divinity, imagination, and power.

By residing directly within the Self (something you learned back in step 1), you can experience greater detachment and clearly observe the fundamental relationship between sentience and energy. See sentience and energy as the divine interplay of your everyday existence, because it is. Everything you do, or do not do, is an interaction between your sentience and the body of energy you have been given to create with. When you wake in the morning, it's your sentience that commands the energy within your physical body to get out of bed and head for work. It's the sentience that commands your energy to process stimuli, which creates thought. The interplay of sentience and energy is tangibly obvious when your physical body is so irreparably damaged that the command of energy you send can't make it to the area you wish to animate, like trying to move when you're paralyzed.

Higher States of Consciousness and Energy Healing

All healing is energy healing. Universal life force, or energy, commonly referred to as prana, exists everywhere, though predominantly in more subtle frequential states outside of the limited perception of the body's five physical senses. Energy healing has been practiced for millions of years. Yes, *millions*.

Similarly, throughout antiquity, shamans would alter their consciousness by raising the electromagnetic frequency of their brain, often through natural substances or chanting and praying, in order to gain access to higher frequencies. The purpose of accessing these higher realms was to glean wisdom, liberation, or a cure. In a heightened state of consciousness or raised awareness, sometimes these shamans would communicate directly with the inherent intelligence of nature itself, such as elementals, plants, mushrooms, and herbs.

There are many ancient texts and recent research that reference beings who could access higher states of consciousness in order to download needed information or to heal individuals or societies. In Lemuria, Atlantis, and ancient Egypt, just to name a few, we refer to those beings as high priests, advanced beings, or even Masters. These individuals were the most respected and revered individuals in their societies. Within nearly all religions and spiritual practices, the achieving of higher intuitive functionality is considered to be a "godly state," or the penultimate state of being, prior to achieving authentic enlightenment.

There needs to be a certain level of purity in order to work in this elevated fashion. Egoic endeavors are the realm of duality, the lower frequencies, and therefore act as anchors or barriers to higher frequential planes of existence and enhanced functionality.

The only impediments you have to the direct connection with your higher consciousness are your misperceptions, misunderstandings, and misidentifications—all of which are the data stream of information that is your egoic identity. All of those phenomena are the past. Whenever you misidentify the Self with something and believe in it, you begin to create a hierarchy of beliefs. This gives that data stream various levels of importance. This importance is how you prioritize your existence and is the weight that sways your already complete consciousness, imbalances your originally pure body of energy, and robs you of your innate freedom. Remember, all thoughts are equal in weightlessness. They are all empty. There is no thought that weighs more than another. You decide which thoughts are important based upon your beliefs and thus give them their weight and sway over your True Self.

You Are Eternally within and Part of the Greater Reality

My experience and understanding is that there is no such thing as actual matter, but rather that everything is simply sentience and energy vibrating at various frequencies.

All existence occupies the same "space" concurrently but is simply not accessible through human sensory perceptions. What you refer to and experience as the physical universe simply consists of sentience and energy vibrating within a range or band of specific frequencies, the overwhelming majority of which are outside the perception of what the physical body is attuned to.

There are a multitude of frequencies, sub-frequencies, sub-sub-frequencies, sub-sub-sub-frequencies (at least seven subs), dimensions, and parallel concurrent versions of everything that make up the multiverse within the Greater Reality. And more. It is an ever-expanding holographic hall of mirrors devised for existence to know itself in totality, which can never actually completely occur. I know your finite mind wants an end point, but it doesn't exist. Certain experiences have a beginning and an end, like an incarnation, but not the experience of existence itself. We all play an integral part in this whether we realize and believe it or not, and even if we don't want to, refuse to, or even don't care to at this moment.

Eventually you will understand this tangibly, not just mentally, and you will be compelled to act with more love and compassion than you can possibly imagine right now. There are meditations that I teach that significantly alter the electromagnetic frequency of your brain, one of which you are about to learn in this chapter, that enable you to experience different planes of existence. Just think of a high-rise building. In order to take the elevator and experience the upper floors, we must raise the electromagnetic frequency of our receiver—the brain. The physical body is attuned to and part of the lowest floors only, but your sentience is attuned to the Architect of all creation.

The creative process itself is a limitless self-generated, self-directed, self-perpetuating, and self-correcting consciousness in and of itself. The Architect/Creator and all of its creations and those creations' creations are eternally creating. Your identification with anything like the physical body, past/future lives, concepts, knowledge, memories, beliefs, expectations, and fears prevents the total freeing of your Self's limitless imagination and ability to perceive beyond the physical senses.

The Chakras and the Human Energy Field

A chakra, which means "spinning wheel of energy," is part of an energetic system that exists for all incarnate life but varies according to form factor, vehicle, or species. Chakras transform both higher- and lower-frequency subtle energies in order to sustain the form and functionality of any body type within the physical universe. This more subtle frequential energy is utilized or metabolized by the chakra system, and this is what sustains the functionality of the life "form," including its organs, systems, body parts, cells, etc. As we deepen our sentience, we will realize it isn't physical food that sustains us but the energies that our chakras metabolize. It's why people can go extremely long periods of time without eating and greatly improve their health through fasting. I talk much more about this and in great detail in the appendix.

Many ancient and holy texts are filled with accounts of mystics, yogis, and Masters who fast and meditate for very long periods of time. It is a discipline and practice only to be undertaken when the Self is deeply understood or when there is a deep desire to do so. Most of us are not ready to work with ourselves in this way. But there are some humans who rarely eat now, and their aging process is significantly reduced and their physical health is optimal. There are centers today that, under the strict supervision of trained doc-tors, help you heal and restore your system for better health through fasting. This further emphasizes that we are sustained energetically through our chakra system. Personally, I have gone weeks at a time consuming only electrolyte and mineral-rich water in order to help restart, restore, and repair my physical body. Again, much more on this in the appendix.

The chakra system runs along hundreds of meridians and cen-ter points called *nadis* that encompass the lowest energetic physi-cal template. There are many books that explore and describe the chakras in great detail, but for our purposes this basic understand-ing will suffice.

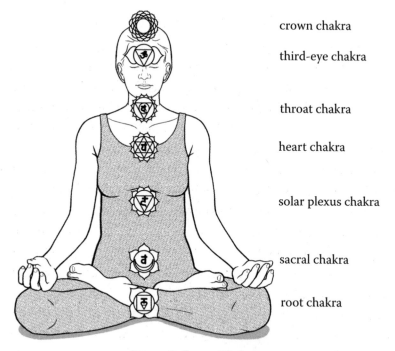

crown chakra

third-eye chakra

throat chakra

heart chakra

solar plexus chakra

sacral chakra

root chakra

Figure 2: Seven Chakras

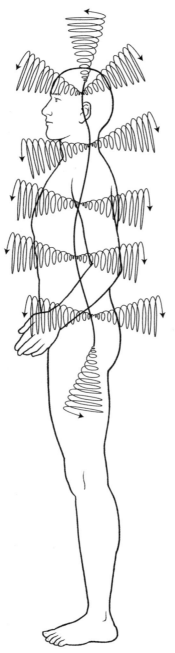

Figure 3: Twelve Chakras

There are seven main chakras associated with the human form (figure 2), although there are actually twelve main chakras that encapsulate the overall chakra system (figure 3) and many, many mini chakras not included in the master twelve. We have one top, or crown, chakra and one bottom, or root, chakra. The middle five chakras have a front and rear chakra for a total of twelve main chakras. Our front chakras work with our intention, and our rear chakras propel us. Think of your rear chakras as the engine at the back of your boat. They are thrusters, or energy boosters, that help us carry out our intention. Our human energy field correlates to specific systems and functionality, as it relates to the physical, emotional, and mental aspects as well as the purely energetic and spiritual. The numbers 3, 7, and 12 relate to the structure of our energy field and, not coincidentally, the structure of our multiverse in an astounding and complete fashion. As above, so below.

The lower three chakras—the root, sacral, and solar plexus—are masculine in nature and predominantly relate to the material or physical world. The top three chakras—the crown, third-eye, and throat chakras—are feminine in nature and predominantly relate to the spiritual world or the realm of higher intuitive functionality and creativity. The fourth chakra, the heart chakra, is the balance between the spiritual and physical planes. Not so coincidentally, as there are no coincidences, this is precisely where your sentience resides, between the heart and the spine. As we mentioned earlier, this is why we always point to the center of our chest and not our head when signifying "me."

When we closely observe our twelve main chakras, we begin to understand the various frequencies that our energy field exists within when incarnate, as well as the "experience of color" associated with various frequential rates.

Many decades ago, Heinrich Rudolf Hertz was the first person to provide conclusive proof of the existence of electromagnetic waves.

Their frequency is measured in Hertz (Hz), which is equal to one cycle per second. Hertz can be measured by an electronic frequency counter, a spectrum analyzer, or an oscilloscope, among many other devices.

1. Our root chakra exists within a frequency of 256 Hz and creates the ocular experience of the color red.

2. Our sacral chakra exists within a frequency of 288 Hz and creates the ocular experience of the color orange.

3. Our solar plexus chakra exists within a frequency of 320 Hz and creates the ocular experience of the color yellow.

4. Our heart chakra exists within a frequency of 352 Hz and creates the ocular experience of the color green.

5. Our throat chakra exists within a frequency of 384 Hz and creates the ocular experience of the color blue.

6. Our third-eye chakra exists within a frequency of 432 Hz and creates the ocular experience of the color indigo.

7. Our crown chakra exists within a frequency of 480 Hz and creates the ocular experience of the color violet.

By listening to tones that vibrate within the frequencies that are associated with various chakras, we help bring the chakras back into a harmonious state by recalibrating them to their natural frequency, or spin rate. What is interesting to note is that the number of petals on the root chakra is 4, on the sacral chakra is 6, on the solar plexus chakra is 10, on the heart chakra is 12, and on the throat chakra is 16, for a total of 48, which corresponds to the 48 nerves in the autonomic nervous system. The crown chakra's main lotus consists of 12 petals (960 total vortices), which corresponds with the 12 cranial nerves. Again, more noncoincidences.

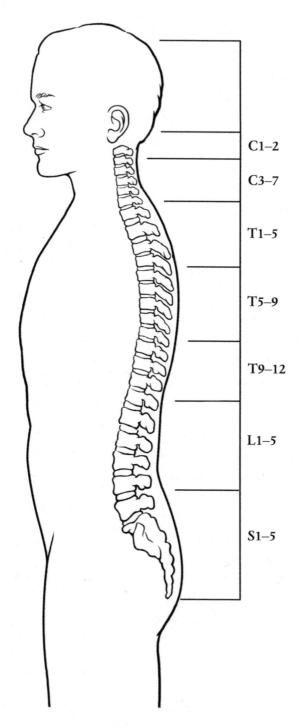

C1–2

C3–7

T1–5

T5–9

T9–12

L1–5

S1–5

Figure 4: Spine and Chakras

In terms of our spine, the root chakra corresponds with L4 and L5 within the vertebrae; the sacral chakra with L1, L2, and L3; the solar plexus chakra with T8, T9, T10, T11, and T12; the heart chakra with T2, T3, T4, T5, T6, and T7; and the throat chakra with C1, C2, C3, C4, C5, C6, C7, and T1 (figure 4).

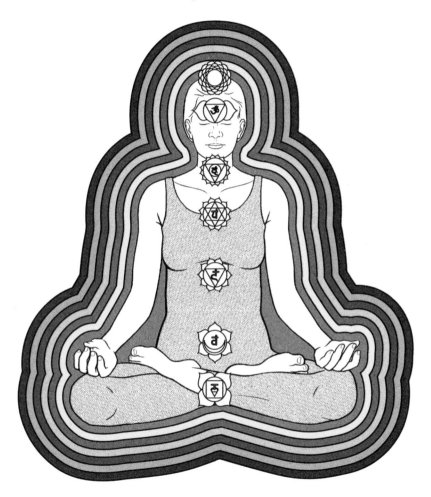

Figure 5: Auric Layers

The subtle bioenergy that radiates from all the chakras forms our auric layers, which are a translation of our energetic templates (figure 5). All of it is one larger system: you. A microcosm of the macrocosm.

Contrary to popular accepted spiritual belief, a person's aura is but a sliver of the energy directly surrounding the Self. The aura is created as a type of "discharge" from the Self. The Self affects all energies, especially the energy closest to it.

The seven main layers of the human energy field (there are ten layers in total) consist of the densest or slowest of frequencies all the way to the lightest or quickest in frequency. These layers are directly related to our traditional system of seven (now we know more accurately, twelve) chakras. Eastern philosophy and medicine have used some of this information for eons. Masters, healers, shamans, mystics, and sages have long accessed these higher frequencies in order to help heal, enlighten, and free themselves as well as their people.

In Eastern medicine, the seven main layers of the human energy field correspond to the seven main chakras as follows:

- The etheric body (physical body) is associated with the root chakra.
- The emotional body (emotions) is associated with the sacral chakra.
- The mental body (thought) is associated with the solar plexus chakra.
- The astral body (soul) is associated with the heart chakra.
- The etheric template (voice) is associated with the throat chakra.
- The celestial body (vision of the soul) is associated with the third-eye chakra.
- The ketheric body (self-realization) is associated with the crown chakra.

Our blueprint and template for optimum health exists within much higher and subtle frequencies. It is my experience that our body of energy exists within the tenth frequency (figure 6), three above the traditional seven-chakra system. Their vibration (and *vibration* is really another word for *information*) cascades down frequentially into our templates. This information—you—continues to express itself and is translated all the way into the lowest frequencies within the physical universe. The result is your physical body. It is only our disharmonious thought patterns through misperceptions, misunderstandings, and misidentifications (the egoic identity) that misprogram our energies and create the programs of ill health. When misidentification is deep enough, this misprogramming is now part of our larger body of energy. This greatly affects the health and expression of the physical body we incarnate into as well as other future incarnations.

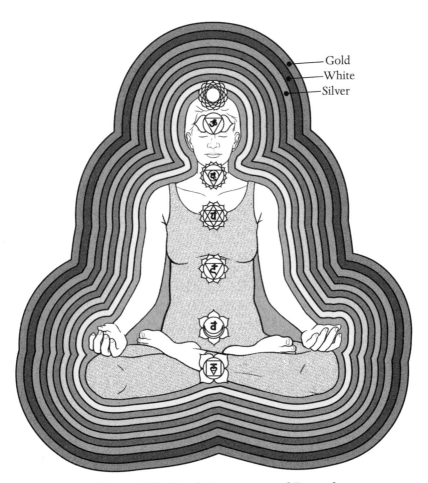

Figure 6: The Tenth Frequency and Beyond

Higher Frequency Bands Are Not Actual Chakras

In actuality, there are twelve total frequency bands that relate to the human energy field, but there are only seven main layers associated with the chakra system of the human form. There are three frequency bands above the crown chakra and one frequency band below the root chakra, which extends about eighteen inches into the earth.

The eighth frequency band is located about one inch above the crown chakra, is gold in color, and represents the transcendence of time. When working with this frequency band, we delve into parallel lives, alternate realities, and communication with our non-incarnate guides and helpers, commonly miscalled angels.

The ninth frequency band is located slightly higher than the eighth and allows one to access the soul's life plan and possible exit points from the current incarnation. It is translucent silvery-white in color. This realm feels very pliable and more ephemeral than tangible or solid.

The tenth frequency band is located about eighteen inches into the earth and connects to the energies of Gaia (earth). It helps to ground us and connect us to the entire natural world.

The eleventh frequency band is located near the outer edge of the human energy field above the ninth frequency band. A powerful healer can use this frequency to realign the etheric templates. This is a realm of pure intention, manipulating a field of patterned energy. It seems to be a mixture of violet, gold, and silver. Definitive and separate representations of color are difficult to distinguish. My understanding is that in the most advanced states of incarnate beingness, one can access this realm, become a conduit, and reopen the pathway for sentience and energy to potentially reanimate a recently lifeless form factor, but only if it is in the life plan of that soul.

The twelfth frequency band exists as the boundary of what we experience as the totality of the individualized soul's energy field and acts as the line of demarcation of where our sense of physicality ends and pure spirit begins. It's a translucent, multicolored realm of light.

It seems to represent the transcendence of any individualized identifications with a physical self or, more specifically, physical incarnation itself. This is where direct communication between the Higher
Self and the incarnate soul can take place, and also, on rare occasion,
what appears to be the possibility of alteration to the incarnate soul
by the Higher Self.

The thirteenth frequency band is a viewing station of the entire
physical universe. It exists as a kind of last stop before we enter the
second full dimension where our current experience of physicality
would no longer exist.

Never Let the Little You (the EMI) Conquer the Big You (the True Self)

What is original to us all is optimum health and incredible longevity.
Once the evolutionary cycle of low-frequency incarnation begins, we
are subject to a lack of tangible self-awareness. This non-holistic way
of living provides sentience the experience of suffering and ill health
through the human experience. Our lack of true self-understanding
then becomes tangibly experienced within our physical body's imbalances. It is our lack of Self-consciousness and what we miscreate due
to this separation, the egoic identity, that destroys any opportunity
for healing, freedom, and self-realization. It's why the ATFHT is revolutionary in its ability to greatly improve the quality of your life as
well as your health on all levels.

Everything that our multi-frequential energy field is exposed to
becomes metabolized by our chakra system. These energies greatly
affect us. The egoic identity lowers our naturally robust energetic
shield. From the egoic identity, belief systems provide the context
for disharmonious thoughts, which create disharmonious emotions,
disharmonious actions, disharmonious behaviors, and disharmonious experiences, including ill health—all of which correlate to the
programming of the false self we have miscreated for ourselves.

You can rebuild and repair your temporary physical body by disempowering the egoic identity program of limitations that controls

it. When you're living in clarity, calmness, connectivity, and communion, meaning observing without finite mental analysis (prejudgment), action takes place. The activation of divine intelligence—our eternal wisdom, unconditional love, and courage to act—is automatically engaged. This uninterrupted, perpetual state of "beingness" automatically realigns and repairs our multi-frequential energy field. This is the definitive state of harmony and healing. Whatever disharmonious energies we have accumulated are transmuted or present themselves so they can be worked with and subsequently reprogrammed, deleted, or harmonized through the various steps of the ATFHT.

You are a perfect and synchronous individualized expression of freedom itself—of divine loving intelligence. It is only when this pure self-awareness misidentifies itself with anything other than its own creator-beingness that subsequent disharmonious thought patterns manifest and throw what is naturally harmonious, free, and perfect out of balance.

Client Example: Hypothyroidism, Neck Injury, Opioid Dependency

Victor is in his early forties and endured a traumatic motorcycle accident causing a severe neck injury. He developed an opioid dependency and debilitating hypothyroidism from a constant overuse of stimulants in order to keep him functional. I met Victor through his wife, who was a patient at the same rehab center as me. She suffered a traumatic brain injury, leaving her incoherent and paralyzed from the waist down. He came to see me at my office with a fairly open mind but with a dwindling energy for himself and his responsibilities.

I asked him how I could help.

"I don't know where to start." Victor's emotions immediately came to the surface, and his eyes began to tear. "Nothing has turned out like I thought it would. My wife and I got injured six years ago on my motorcycle only a few years after we got married. She is not mentally aware and is in a wheelchair, as you know, and I damaged two vertebrae in my neck. I'm in constant pain and always exhausted. My mind is slipping because of all the meds I take. I'm a mess all the time, but I have to take care of her, and it's killing me."

He needed to admit this to someone else so he could stop lying to himself. His suffering, as well as his wife's, had become unbearable for him. He caught a quick glance of my old wheelchair and walker still in the corner of my office behind me. "I know you know what I'm talking about, RJ. You understand what it's *really* like."

That was it for him. This bull of a man completely broke down. He'd been suffering from not just his own pain but his wife's too. His anger at not having the life he had imagined, at not seeing any improvement in himself or his unreachable wife, was eating him alive. I said nothing because, at that moment, words were not the cure. He stared into my eyes, looking for an answer to the end of his suffering. I could feel it. This was a powerful man who has been brought to his knees. Maybe he was ready to listen with the ears of his heart.

Victor looked deeply at me, searching for an end to his misery. "How did *you* get better?"

That was not the right question. I remained silent but hid nothing.

"Can you help me?"

That's what I needed to hear. "I will help you on one condition," I said. He stopped wiping his eyes and sat up straighter.

I commanded all of his attention by giving him all of mine. "No more new tears over the past or future. You must be fully present in the now for true energetic healing to begin. If you can make that promise to yourself and me, I will help you. Think very carefully before you answer."

Victor never expected that he would be presented with this challenge, just as he never expected the challenges in his life. He would have to leave both his expectations and his ruminations behind in order for me to really show him how to heal himself.

"I can do nothing about the past, and neither can you. The future doesn't exist. If you aren't really done with them, then there is obviously nothing new to discuss."

He sat silent. This was his opportunity to move out of suffering and into new possibilities, but he had to make that conscious choice. I do not work with those who aren't ready to work directly with the Self. I could feel his resoluteness. He put his handkerchief away and said, "No more new tears for the past or future. I promise." And with that, he nodded in recognition of his own promise.

I couldn't keep the smile from my face, no matter how tough I was being with him.

"Wonderful. Now I am talking to the Real You. Welcome back. I'm going to teach you how to direct the repair and healing of your neck and thyroid."

I guided Victor to a state of higher consciousness that one can access only through a specific meditation, which you will learn at the end of this chapter. Once the brain had been attuned to a much faster vibratory rate, we could begin reconstructing and repairing his damaged energy field, which includes the physical body. Tangibly speaking, significantly higher frequencies feel the opposite of what you might expect, meaning they feel infinitely more spacious even though energy is actually moving much faster than in our lower frequencies. Our brain is simply not naturally attuned to these higher frequencies and therefore has no frame of reference. Hence, it feels empty and blissfully calm. I walked him through the precise way to work most efficiently in regard to the reconstruction of the physical body.

After a few weeks of consistently performing this healing meditation, Victor began to feel less and less pain in his neck. He could feel his metabolism becoming more balanced through working on his thyroid. After six weeks of consistent application of step 4 of the ATFHT, he reported a massive reduction in neck pain. He called my office to schedule another session but wanted to speak with me before he did.

"RJ, I can turn my head from side to side and even shrug my shoulders and it doesn't hurt. I haven't been able to do that since the accident. I haven't taken a single opioid in a month either. I feel alive again!"

With his new understanding of how self-healing really works, his thyroid became much healthier. He felt a much steadier flow of natural energy and could perform all his daily tasks without always feeling exhausted. He simply gave his thyroid what it needed. Victor relayed to me that the moment he gave up entirely on reliving the past and projecting its fear-based future, he felt truly empowered and energized. He knew he would be able to repair and heal himself once he had the proper blueprint to follow. He came to see me one last time.

"I understand now. My wife and I gave ourselves these challenges so we could help each other learn acceptance with grace and courage. I wasn't doing that because all I did was live in the past or worry about the future. The moment I decided I would never shed a new tear over the past or future, I gave myself a new possibility: healing. I get it now."

Step 4 Core Exercise:
Healing Meditation to Command
Creator Consciousness

This is the meditation that I taught Victor. This should be done daily and can be done multiple times a day. Whatever specific system, organ, body part, nerve, or cells need repair and healing, you can target and solely rebuild that specific area while in this state of consciousness whenever needed.

You may find it useful to record yourself narrating this meditation. Turn on wordless higher-frequency tones that complement this journey and speak softly but with conviction. Alternately, you could ask a like-minded friend to lead you through it, and then take turns leading each other. Let's meditate now, together.

Sit on the floor or on a mat in the lotus position, if possible. If this is not comfortable, sit in a flat-back chair, with your back straight and your feet firmly planted on the ground. Now comfortably rest your hands on your upper thighs, palms up. Tilt your head slightly downward, keeping your jaw loose and your tongue relaxed in the back of your mouth like a clam in the back of its shell. Close your eyes. Using the diaphragm, take a deep breath in through the nose and exhale out the mouth. Belly breathing directly connects conscious attention with our sentience. Take two more deep, full breaths. You may feel the mind already becoming still. Remember to keep your jaw loose and your tongue relaxed. Just breathe normally now from the belly. Let the mind settle down. If a thought pops into your head, just say to yourself, "That's just a thought, that's not me," and let it go. Breathe. Repeat this until the mind is no longer grabbing for thoughts to sustain itself. Experience your own exquisite inner silence and stillness.

Free yourself from analyzing or responding to bodily sensations. Let the body do what it will. Just observe it. You are not the physical body. Let go of the misidentification with it. If any sensation arises, simply say to yourself, "That's just a sensation, that's not me," and let it go. Once the mind is still, the physical body will feel hollow and empty, as though there is only a faint outline of it. Gently stay right there. Breathe. You are now consciously aware of what you eternally are: formless, free, and unconditioned. You are creator awareness given energy to create as you deem fit. Breathe. No more physical body or human mind. Simply an etheric, translucent form.

Imagine yourself standing on a deserted road in the middle of absolutely nowhere. You slowly begin to realize that before you is a huge airplane hangar with a single metal door. Slowly move your awareness toward the door. Set your intention to open the door. Open it *now*. Before you is the most technically advanced spacecraft imaginable. Take in its otherworldly design and sheer perfection. There is absolutely nothing this craft cannot do, and it was built and designed specifically for you. Move your awareness to the entrance of your perfect craft. Set your intention to open the entry hatch. Do it *now*. Bring your awareness inside your craft. It is a technological marvel beyond anything known to humankind. It responds directly to your every thought, emotion, and intention. Its intelligent system is specifically aligned to your vibrational signature. Its singular purpose is to afford your awareness safe travel to anywhere.

Bring your awareness to the viewing screen and place your translucent hands on the control panel. Your craft will instantly and always respond to your every intention. Once you have acclimated yourself to your new craft, get ready to transcend the lower frequencies of the physical universe. You are aware that momentarily we are going to jettison up the frequencies and dimensions of the multiverse into the higher frequencies of existence itself, well beyond space and time, where there is no static or fixed form to anything. The ether is pure potential that immediately yields to the power of your imagination. In this realm, Intelligent Energy is free of all limitations. The power of our creative intention instantaneously shapes this pure environment. Our desired reality is instantly co-created. This realm is *real*.

Send the intention to skyrocket straight up the frequencies *now*. Feel yourself, your vibration, nearly lifting off your seat. Gravity is being shed. You feel the waves of energy cascading down around your head and shoulders as you exit this frequency. Count to yourself slowly as you ascend: 3, 4, 5 … 10. (We start at 3, as we currently reside within the 3rd frequency.) You feel the lightness of being, the emptiness of non-physicality, the freedom of higher frequencies. Each moment of acceleration up the frequencies makes you feel lighter, calm, almost euphoric. Continue slowly counting to yourself: 11, 12, 13 … 20. Feel the ascension up the frequencies all over your translucent form. Keep ascending, higher and higher. You are eternally safe and protected in your craft. It was built and designed only for you. 21, 22, 23 … 39. Keep ascending: 40, 41, 42 … 50.

You are leaving the association and use of the physical body and its analytical mind. It is the only way to transcend it. Once you start to become aware of the liberation from the human experi-ence, send the intention to slow your craft down. Acclimate your-self to this purer, truer state of beingness. Ease down on your hyper speed until you hover at a complete standstill. Your craft responds instantaneously to your intention. Just stay here. Let yourself adjust to the higher frequencies of existence. Once you are fully adjusted and ready, set your intention to step outside your craft. There is no gravity or the need for it. Your pure intention sustains and takes you wherever your attention goes. Step outside *now*. Take in the envi-ronment. Feel the supremely high frequency. What does this envi-ronment feel like? Look like? Just be with it without judging it.

Only when inspired to do so, set your intention to bring Intelli-gent Energy that is available everywhere in this environment to you. You are a powerful creator. Shape and form these intelligent ener-gies into a pristine and perfect holographic version of your health-iest self. Let your higher imagination and its pure creative energy flow through you. Build yourself anew—every single body part, every internal system, every organ, every nerve, muscle, and cell. Create yourself down to the tiniest divine and perfect detail. Once complete, place your perfect "you" just in front of you. Do it *now*. This new version of yourself is the perfect original design of opti-mal health. Feel that it was your imagination that created this per-fect and pristine you. Every system, every organ, every bone, every nerve pathway, every beat of your heart, and every cell have all been constructed in perfect, divine alignment, pulsing with immense life force. And you can see it and feel it.

This is precisely how you were originally designed before you were ever born. The design of the human form is an expression of a supreme loving intelligence, and you can now fully experience its true majesty in front of you. You *are* this majesty. Feel the divine, perfect expression that you are. It is You.

Through your unstoppable intention, bring this holographic image of perfection right before you. Bring your divine creation, your perfect you, *into you* and completely merge with it *now*. Unite once again with your perfection. Completely. Utterly. In totality. Surrender. It is your destiny. It is You. Feel the divine energies surging through your body, all of your systems, all of your organs, all of your cells, every proton, neutron, and electron charged with the light of Source. It is repairing you, aligning you, renewing you, healing you. Feel it now. You are reborn new once again.

Next, set your intention to return to your craft. Do it *now*. Awareness (you) recognizes that it exists within a perfectly regenerated and pristine form. Sit down in your control seat. Place your new translucent hands on the control panel and set your intention to descend the frequencies. Do it *now*. Feel the wave of energies all over you as you slowly descend into the slower and denser frequencies. 50, 49, 48 ... 40. Let your consciousness adjust to your new body and the dropping of the frequencies. 39, 38, 37 ... 30. Feel the waves of energy all around you. 29, 28, 27, 26 ... 13. Bring your craft back into physical reality. 12, 11, 10, 9, 8 ... 3. Once you have adjusted back to this realm, set your intention for your craft to land. Do it *now*.

Set your intention to open your spacecraft door and step outside onto solid ground. Do it *now*. Bring your awareness and translucent perfect new body into the deserted airplane hangar and command the entire structure to dematerialize. Do it *now*. You are back in your home now. Breathe. Open your eyes. Take a drink of water to ground yourself. Enjoy and utilize the profound energetic reattunement, reconstruction, and regeneration of your form. Repeat this meditation daily as needed.

❄ ❄ ❄

Master this meditation. Keep using the spaceship until you can rebuild yourself whenever you need to. Realize that the personalized spaceship is a metaphor for your physical body. Your body is the perfect vessel that was built just for you and responds to your every intention. The spaceship is your permission slip to ascend the frequencies and dimensions and heal yourself.

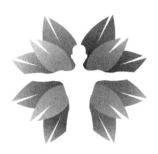

Step 5

Channel Intelligent Energy into the Body

The higher frequencies or realms of existence consist of "Intelligent Energy" that naturally harmonizes and repairs the energy that exists in lower frequencies. By applying step 5, we learn how to access this ever-present and endlessly available Intelligent Energy for ourselves in order to repair and heal our larger body of energy. This understanding and its application are the bedrock principles of the energy healing modality known as Reiki. Step 5 involves channeling Intelligent Energy into the body through the crown chakra.

Intelligent Energy, as you may recall, is energy that vibrates at various frequencies outside of physical sensory perception. Intelligent Energy, or free energy, exists everywhere, perpetually, but we usually don't recognize its existence, let alone understand how to use it. Nikola Tesla is a rare example of someone who did.

In this step you will learn how to use Intelligent Energy to repair and heal your body with energy. There are countless studies of sound, light, electromagnetic pulses, and other practices being used to aid and accelerate the healing and repair of physical and emotional trauma. For instance, the remarkable results of hyperbaric chambers, which increase the amount of oxygen to greatly enhance healing and recovery, are well documented, but they are insignifi-cant compared to the healing properties of Intelligent Energy. The most powerful Intelligent Energy exists in higher frequencies, and its inherent function is to repair, or, more accurately, harmonize, through the reprogramming of disharmonious energies that vibrate at lower frequencies.

For example, when done properly, the Reiki master harnesses their intention using higher frequential energy, or what has been commonly referred to as the Universal Life Force, to aid in the repair and healing of people, animals, and even locations and objects. The master's level of sentience, power, and purity of intent directly correlates with the ability to access, commandeer, and channel more energy of a higher vibratory rate that repairs and heals all that vibrates in lower frequen-cies, including the astral, physical, emotional, and mental bodies. The more you know your immortal Self tangibly and experientially, not conceptually or emotionally, the greater access you have to the vast-ness of the Greater Reality, and the more potent a healer you become.

Intelligent Energy can repair, harmonize, and reprogram our total body of energy all the way down to the lower frequencies of the physical universe, which includes the physical body. Think of Intel-ligent Energy like putting high-grade fuel in your car, or eating the best organic, non-GMO food, or ingesting the strongest and purest medical marijuana tinctures.

Everything Is Frequency, Energy, and Vibration

Everything is frequency (environment), energy (potentiality), and vibration (information). Energy, as we have discussed, vibrates at different frequencies housed in dimensional constructs within the same space. Through my own direct experience utilizing my last twenty-five years of higher consciousness exploration and impossi-ble healing, it is my understanding that roughly 97 percent of fre-quential states and dimensional constructs are well outside the range that our five physical senses can perceive. Not so coincidentally yet again, that is nearly the same percentage of DNA that we have no tangible understanding of. DNA is the physical representation and tangible experience of humanity's past and present. DNA will also adapt to the limitless capabilities of sentience as we consciously recognize and work with more and more of the immortal Self.

As we work directly with our Total Self through the ATFHT, we accrue or deepen our sentience, which subsequently unlocks more and more of our DNA. I utilized this understanding tangibly in order to bring myself back to life. This is the evolution of consciousness as it relates to healing.

We know that water, always expressed as H_2O, exists as a liquid, solid, steam, and vapor. The less dense or solid the state, the faster its vibratory rate, which is why we can see ice and water, steam barely, but not vapor. Once it leaves the frequency of our perception, it's invisible to us, but it still exists and remains H_2O. The higher frequencies and dimensions are right here in the same space, just like the unseen water vapor. You cannot perceive higher frequencies and dimensions with ordinary sensory perceptions, but not being able to perceive things like vapor, microwaves, radio waves, or purple ultraviolet rays doesn't mean they're not there. The same applies to the Self when someone leaves this world.

Everything that touches ice tends to bind or stick to it because ice is water (H_2O) in its slowest and densest vibratory state. Place your glove or a cup on a block of ice and it will freeze to it. The opposite also holds true when H_2O is in a much higher vibratory state of existence, like as water vapor. Nothing can adhere to it. The same holds true for you, my friends. Raise your vibration by vanquishing your egoic identity and your body of energy becomes more diffused and higher in frequency, making illness very difficult to stick to you.

As you ascend the frequencies while still incarnate, you allow your sentience to operate beyond the limitations of the physical senses and the intellect. You begin to experience different levels of sentient energies, some that are embodied or incarnate, as well as frequential states of existence beyond what the physical body is attuned to. In order to perceive and experience these higher states and what exists within them, you must already exist within these frequencies and environments. It sounds like a catch-22, but it's not.

In order for energy to exist and vibrate within higher frequencies, that energy must be more aware and intelligent, because the entire environment is more consciously aware of itself. As we go up in frequency, the inherent awareness and functionality of that sentience and energy that vibrates in accordance with it does as well. Just like when you turn on the hot tub, everything in it gets warmer.

Let's go back to the deep-sea diver, who must wear a diving bell in order to work hundreds of feet deep within the water. As the person descends, they have the experience of less and less awareness, functionality, and mobility as the pressure increases. The diver wouldn't be able to function at all without being inside the diving bell.

When your Higher Self/Totality desires to experience the dense, slow vibration of the lower frequencies within the physical universe, it projects an individualized unit of itself: You, a Total Self. It needs a vehicle that can operate at this frequency, just like the diver needs a diving bell in order to survive and function. The Total Self's diving bell is the physical body. The body is always and must be attuned to the range of frequential vibrations within its local environment in order to function. Mistakenly and tragically, we limit our awareness only to what the physical body is attuned to via the physical senses. This creates the egoic identity and its finite little mind, because physical sensory perceptions are the extremely limited data stream that creates and perpetually feeds the intellect.

Through meditation, we raise the electromagnetic frequency of the receiver and projector of reality—the brain—to reach these higher frequencies within our sentient Self-awareness and gain greater understanding, mobility, functionality, and access to the Intelligent Energy that exists within this higher frequential environment. Intrinsically, this energy is more "intelligent" because it is not bound by the limitations of a denser, slower, lower frequential state of self-existence or environment.

All physical environments, including Earth, are specific locations within universal space where energy vibrates at an extremely slow rate. Each location is a frequency, which we call a reality or an environment. The lower frequencies of the physical universe afford your sentience the temporary experience of solidity and therefore physicality. This experience of physicality is the opposite of your sentience's naturally higher frequential and dimensional state of being and location.

Identification and the Impact of Your Energy Body

Your sentience *knows* what I'm saying to be true, but the egoic identity—the fear-based, low-frequency human mind that you may misidentify with—will not allow acceptance of its own transitory existence because it needs your life force to continue its temporary existence.

Disharmony and disease are the spoiled fruit born of misidentification. Everything other than the Self is a belief. From beliefs, misidentification often takes the expression of trapped fear, anger that has affected healthy energy flow, unfulfilled expectations, a pattern of harmful thoughts, repeated negative feelings directed at oneself, feeling sorry for oneself, or a lack of self-worth that leads to poor choices in terms of nutrition, relationships, friends, and experiences. These experiences can also manifest as conditions such as anxiety, addiction, autoimmune disease, depression, cancer, heart disease, diabetes, complications from surgery, and chronic severe pain. This list could go on for pages. All of these experiences live within the multi-frequential layers of our energy field that permeate and subsequently misprogram our physical body, causing ill health and disease. All are attachments born of misidentification. Think of Spider-Man shooting a web and connecting himself to something. This is what a misidentification is like. You have become attached to something you are not. This limits your imagination, innate freedom, and natural harmonic balance. Instead, you are now attached to something outside the Self. This causes great energetic harm and a subsequent poor quality of life. Sometimes exterior phenomena are thrust upon us, whether it's a belief or a virus, but it is always our lack of self-awareness that prevents the proper nonengagement and robust defense against it. From a weakened state due to the disharmonious egoic identity, we continually attach and identify rather than having our powerful energetic drawbridge of non-identification up, preventing the infiltration of foreign invaders.

Remember, the five physical senses only interpret electrical impulses within our local frequential environment. Those electrical impulses are received in the brain, which is in the water, in the dark, and encased in bone, and then our mind creates this "reality." It's an extremely limited coded construct, and that is why your egoic identity is a program of limitations as well. The challenge is to be the Real You in the harshest of environments… and share your divinity, talent, and compassion with the world creatively, uniquely, as only you can.

This is good, this is bad, I like this, I don't like that, this is right, this is wrong. These are simply individualized experiences or interpretations. Currently there are nearly eight billion people on this planet, and every single one of them thinks what they do is right. What precisely are those decisions based on? Your conceptualized, belief-based, miscreated false identity. When you divorce your egoic identity, what it produces—separation, delusion, illusion, and suffering—begins to lift. Then you are tangibly free. Liberation has occurred. Wisdom, love, and power are now fully online… the Real You.

We don't have a total understanding of Self. We lack a conscious understanding of our energetic body and what's embedded within it, cumulatively, lifetime after lifetime. This directly correlates to the level or tangible experience of health, freedom, divinity, and ability to create without limitations during our incarnations.

Non-clarity and attachment is a self-fulfilling cycle of ill health, disharmony, disease, dysfunction, decrepitude, and demise. This non-clarity and attachment is then tangibly experienced through our suffering and expressed within our body of energy. Liberation frees the

Self from all attachments and restores clarity. As awareness unfolds and recognizes itself, ill health and a poor quality of life become unnecessary. Greater self-awareness would prevent the game of victim/perpetrator from even being played.

Many health practitioners are coming to the realization that inflammation is the cause of ill health. The false self gets "triggered" or inflamed because its beliefs about itself have been threatened. When who you think you are and how you feel about yourself and the world are not being validated, you take this external stimulus that is not in agreement with your sense of self "personally" and you become upset. On a deeper level, the transient egoic-identity programming is the True Self's inflamed, overcompensating, disconnected, fear-based reactionary state due to incarnating into our low-frequency environment. All of this non-clarity, suffering, and ill health is beneath your immortal perfection.

Upon your greater self-awareness and liberation, you stop taking things personally, because there is no egoic identity filter getting in the way of your inner peace, freedom, acceptance, wisdom, love, and power within. By utilizing the steps of the ATFHT, whatever is trapped within your multi-frequential energy field can be worked with, transmuted, and released. The false identity is now gone, and with no fulcrum of misidentification in place, nothing is held on to, including the concepts, beliefs, expectations, thoughts, emotions, fears, memories, traumas, and experiences that manifest ill health programs to begin with. Once this state of being is normalized, you can truly repair, heal, and transcend all that is not original to you.

As you free your Self, you will realize the universe has perfected its programming; it endlessly supports your imagination so you can perpetually learn about yourself while it simultaneously learns about itself through your creativity.

The Crown Chakra

The highest frequency most commonly associated with your energetic body while incarnate is that which correlates to the seventh, or crown, chakra. We pay special attention to this chakra in step 5. It is also the chakra associated with true wisdom and enlightenment. There have been many artistic interpretations of halos above the heads of self-realized beings like Christ and Buddha. The halo represents the fully illuminated and activated crown chakra. Another self-realized being, St. Germain, has been described as the embodiment of the Violet Flame, which is the color associated with the crown chakra that signifies self-mastery—the ability to transmute all disharmony into harmony.

When we open our crown chakra, we put ourselves in position to access our higher consciousness. Many people talk about "downloads" of higher knowledge or information that they get through their activated crown chakra. The act of accessing is a "no mind" state. All imagination occurs within your higher consciousness, well beyond the low-frequency machinations of the finite mind. Athletes call this being "in the zone." I recall as a little kid hearing Larry Bird and Magic Johnson saying they could "sense" what was happening on the basketball court, which allowed them to make no-look passes or anticipate what someone was about to do. This allowed them to thwart their opponents' advances seemingly ahead of time.

Artists throughout history have termed our contemporary no-mind state as "the muse being upon them." Whether you think of yourself as an artist or not, you know what it's like to experience this state of oneness and connectivity that transcends thought whenever you lose yourself in a creative endeavor such as dancing, athletics, playing a musical instrument, gardening, writing, painting, singing, cooking, channeling, etc. We lose our sense of a separate self in the act of pure creativity. What we actually lose is the limiting programming of the egoic identity, and therefore no thought is experienced. You are a creation of creation itself, and you experience a transcendental state of oneness when in the act of being creative. You experience the awakening of your divine intelligence and your true power as an immortal creator being in this state. This is meditation.

Client Example: Blood Toxicity, Severe Pain, and Limited Functionality

After attending my introduction to meditation class and doing a few private sessions with me, Maurice decided that he wanted to learn how to heal himself.

A sixth-degree black belt in Tae Kwon Do and Hapkido with over thirty-five years of strict dedication to his martial arts, Maurice was suffering from a rare blood toxicity condition as well as severe pain and very limited functionality in his shoulder, knees, and ankles from multiple surgeries.

Maurice was not only having trouble physically but was stuck in his spiritual evolution as well. He had hit a wall and was unable to take his level of self-awareness and meditation further. This caused him great frustration. Maurice needed to break free from the self-imposed constraints of his current spiritual standstill, recover from his rare blood disorder, alleviate his constant pain, and improve his physical mobility.

His powerful focus simply needed to be harnessed and properly directed. This would allow his already advanced sentience to regain dominion over the egoic identity's program of limitations and direct the repair and healing of his damaged body. While extremely intense, he had a very good sense of humor, was even-keeled, and had fine-tuned his power of self-control, self-discipline, and concentration through his extensive martial arts training. I knew he had a tremendous amount of sentience and energy with which to work. I explained that if intention is clear, specific, and pure, and we powerfully harness the will, disharmony will be harmonized. Maurice understood this immediately.

During our third session, we spoke about the distance, or detachment, required to disengage from body consciousness and thought itself (things we covered in step 1). Both are prerequisites for potently transmuting and transcending disharmony. I explained step 5, which is channeling Intelligent Energy into the body through the crown chakra.

"How fast is it supposed to work?" he asked.

"By focusing on any anticipated result, rather than the process, you're allowing the egoic mind to take over with expectations. Expectations are limitations and have nothing to do with now. Anything other than the clarity and communion of now are the meanderings of the egoic identity, and they prevent efficacy."

He nodded, but I didn't sense that he tangibly understood.

I explained further. "You're losing focus of the moment-to-moment attention and intention required to empty yourself. Both are necessary components of surrender. You must first surrender to harness creativity purposely and powerfully."

"What should I expect to see with my third eye?" he asked.

I needed to get him to truly understand. "Who is it that cares about what is seen or not seen? That's the egoic identity talking."

"Right. I understand." Maurice's mind wasn't done though, cleverly posing the question, "But what does it feel like? So I know if I'm doing it right."

"Focus on the moment, Maurice. Allow each successive *now* to flow through you. Simply do what you experientially know to be true, each moment, and expect no results. Now you are most powerful because you are clear and free."

I could see his sentience trying to break through the human eyes of misperception. To nail down the point, I said, "Do not let the mind grasp at anything."

The sentience within him recognized the instruction of truth and something shifted. He sat up straighter. "I get it now."

"Now, find out what Intelligent Energy feels like by doing the 'Channel Intelligent Energy through the Crown Chakra' exercise [at the end of this chapter] and tell me about it next time we speak."

"Okay," he said. "I trust you."

"Trust *yourself*."

When Maurice arrived for his next appointment, he looked like he was trying to contain his excitement, even though his energy was already announcing it to the world.

A huge smile spread across his face. "I did exactly as you instructed. I opened my crown chakra and envisioned an endless waterfall of Intelligent Energy. Through my intention, I commanded the energy to pour down into my crown. I could feel tingles all around the top of my head. It was like a delicate, pleasant electric current. Almost like how an herbal tea runs down your throat, just more subtle. The image you gave me of the never-ending waterfall was perfect. It felt amazing."

"Fantastic," I said. "I'm not surprised at all at your immediate success. See how it only matters that you directly experience it for yourself, without any expectations getting in the way?"

"Yes. I would have been reaching instead of making it happen myself."

"Exactly. Reaching is worthless. It disempowers you. Command comes from within and empowers you."

"I see that now," he said, "but I wasn't able to move the energy throughout my body as well as I know I'm capable of doing. I need to work on that part."

"It's not difficult. It just takes the proper focus, which is really the diligence of gentle tenacity. Simply follow your attention and intention to move the Intelligent Energy through your crown and into your heart and belly. Remember, if it isn't simple, it's a mental exercise. Stay away from that."

He nodded. "I will. I want to heal myself. I know I can do it."

"Of course you can. Command it."

As we practiced together, Maurice began to realize that the only reason he was not fully directing the energy to where it needed to go for his healing was due to a drop in the conviction that he was doing the latter part correctly. His attention and intention wavered due to doubt.

I asked him, "Does it make sense that you can feel yourself channeling higher frequential energy into your crown but then decide that somehow you can't simply move it to where it needs to go?"

"When you say it like that..."

"How else should I say it? It's foolishness." Maurice is a highly skilled martial arts master and very sentient. He needed no coddling whatsoever. "You tell me when you want to get serious about healing yourself and then we can continue."

He lifted his head and looked at me. "I'm ready."

"Of course you are. Now *show* yourself that you are and *do it*."

Maurice performed step 5 repeatedly over the next five weeks and then the moment of truth arrived. Prior to this point, his blood toxicity disorder had been going on for many, many years with no improvement whatsoever. He and his medical team had been reduced to simply managing his disorder instead of curing it.

Following this practice, blood tests showed a "miraculous and drastic" improvement. Maurice had to explain to his doctor that he had been diligently working on healing himself, since his new results transcended what years of prescribed treatment had achieved. Not only was his blood much healthier, but the dexterity and strength in his knees and ankles improved as well. These results also far exceeded those of the physical therapy he had been doing and without the pain and soreness associated with the prescribed exercises. Maurice is now much healthier and progressing well with his spiritual development.

Step 5 Core Exercise: Channel Intelligent Energy through the Crown Chakra

In order to keep operating at your highest healing potential, clearly, succinctly, and in the present tense, restate your intention in terms of what specifically you are trying to achieve in regard to your health. You can restate your intention prior to any or all of the steps as needed.

As stated previously, the seventh chakra, or crown chakra, is the highest frequential energy transformer most directly associated with the human form. By opening the crown chakra, we can take in the Intelligent Energy that's vibrating at the seventh frequency band

(and above), which is a higher and more potent frequency than the energy that our six other main chakras are metabolizing.

Part 1: Receive Energy

- Firmly but gently state your intention to channel highly powerful Intelligent Energy through your open crown chakra and onto whatever area of your body needs healing.

- Imagine a circle of light, or halo, just above your head, like the ones that are in many paintings of saintly or enlightened beings. The crown chakra, like all chakras, can fully extend about nine inches beyond the body, depending on one's ability to work with the chakras. As a refresher, the chakras are shaped like funnels or cones. Our front chakras spin clockwise to take in and metabolize energy, while our rear chakras spin counterclockwise and expel energy like a thruster, propelling us based upon our intention. The thin, pointed end of the funnel connects with the spine and the wider, open end points outward, extending from the body. You can open and extend your crown chakra by focusing your attention on the area just above and around the top of your head.

- Close your eyes and envision the cone-shaped chakra just above your head. Imagine yourself extending and opening this chakra like you would open an umbrella.

- Imagine what it feels like as you do this. Trust that your focused attention and unwavering intention are all that is needed to accomplish this.

- Gently place the tip of your index finger on the very top of your head. Just like in step 1, bring all your attention and focus to the sensation of touch on the top of your head. Remain there.

- Then reach out from inside your head and touch your fingertip. You will feel like the top of your head is opening up, because energetically that is exactly what is happening. You are opening your crown chakra. Keep all your focus and attention right there. At a certain point, you will begin to feel tingling around the top of your head. Keep going. When your crown chakra is open and fully extended, it may feel like someone literally lifted off the top of your head, like removing a tight baseball cap.

- Once you have fully opened and extended your crown chakra, imagine a never-ending waterfall of healing Intelligent Energy cascading down into it. Notice what color the water is.

- Fix your attention and intention on channeling this limitless waterfall of Intelligent Energy through your open and extended crown chakra.

- In your mind's eye, see yourself commanding the Intelligent Energy to flow into and through your crown chakra using your intention. Trust that this is being accomplished.

- Feel the Intelligent Energy experientially. Now it is *known*. The tingling and energy around the top of your head may be unlike anything you've ever felt before. That's a great indicator that you're channeling Intelligent Energy through your crown chakra.

- Gently bring this flowing Intelligent Energy down through your body to whatever area needs repair. See your physical body as just a hollow balloon outline holding a body of energy, because at its true essence it is.

- Set the intention to keep your crown chakra fully open and extended, with never-ending and omnipotent Intelligent Energy continually pouring into it.

- Direct the Intelligent Energy to go wherever it is needed.

- Maintain an unwavering focus on the cascading, healing, and omnipotent Intelligent Energy endlessly pouring through your crown chakra, and feel its current of healing energy going through your hollow body of energy.

- Close your eyes and see what this healing Intelligent Energy actually looks like as it pours through your crown and fills the area of your body that is affected by disharmony. See it and feel it. Your tangible experience of doing this is your meditation. Maintain your resoluteness, and you will experience tactile confirmation of your intention.

When channeling Intelligent Energy through your crown chakra, experiment and discover what's most effective for your own healing. Don't limit or doubt yourself in any way. Tangibly experience it for yourself so you have direct confirmation. Imagine, see, and feel it.

Part 2: Give Energy

It is my experience that an endless waterfall of cascading, healing, omnipotent Intelligent Energy is a good visual for the mind to start with. Some Reiki masters channel their version of Intelligent Energy through their crown chakra and then out their heart chakra or through the mini chakras in the center of their palms and onto their intended recipient, sometimes including themselves.

With practice, you can do this too by directing this healing, omnipotent Intelligent Energy to exit through your heart chakra or palm chakras and onto whatever body part, organ, or internal system you fix your intention upon. Place your attention upon your heart chakra or your palm chakras as your exit point for the channeled energy. Use your intention and the finger touch exercise to open whichever chakras you wish to utilize, just as you did to open your crown chakra. You will feel the opening and expanding of these chakras. Through intention, rotate them in the opposite direction to allow the current of energy to pour right through them instead of into them. See it in your mind's eye and tangibly experience it. It may help to play a video of a waterfall so that the sound enhances your meditation. While in my hospital bed, I would perform this technique with my palm chakras. I'd place my hands about two to three inches above my intestines, bladder, feet, and thyroid many times a day and channel Intelligent Energy into them for repair and healing.

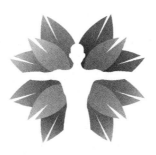

Step 6

Turn Off the Program of Illness

Illness is the tangible experience of disharmony (misprogrammed energy). By accessing the higher frequencies where the building blocks of our form and function exist, we learn to apply step 6 to literally turn off the program of illness we are running.

A Piece of the Ego Identity Limitation Program You Are Running Is Illness Itself

The reason the mind constantly wants more and more information is because it doesn't tangibly know anything. It's simply an electronic receiver (translation medium) and storage facility (memory) of physical sensory perceptions.

See the relationship between the perpetually ravenous, incomplete ego and how the finite mind is always seeking more and more information. That is because both do not authentically know anything. Herein lies a key to better health and a greater quality of life. Gain dominion over your life force for repair and healing instead of squandering it on outward pursuits, including the delusion that health lies outside of you. Diagnosis and illness all belong to personhood, the egoic mind, the outer body of energies. Healing resides at the core of your sentience-directed life force. Remember, what is original to you is absolute. It is perpetual, immortal, and renewable perfection—which exists prior to thought, emotion, the body, and even the evolutionary cycle itself. The Self is immortal. The energy you used to create your egoic identity and its program of limitations is the same energy you will harness to repair and heal.

It is the *same energy within you* that you use to form the thought "I can do this" or "I can't do this." It's the same life force energy. You either mis-qualify the energy by running it through your EMI limitation program or harness it where it starts through limitless imagination. Just as the egoic identity is a limitation program that can be turned off by not feeding it your life force, so too can the program of illness be turned off.

Turn Off the Program of Illness

When we're in a harmonized and balanced state, we don't focus our attention upon things that don't promote harmony and balance. We stop putting unhealthy foods, drinks, or any other "in-formation" into our system. We choose not to seek out stimuli (experiences, information, and people) that are disharmonious. While in this harmonized and balanced state, our entire body of multi-frequential energy naturally fights off invading disharmonious free radicals.

Your sentience, when accessed directly, commands your RNA, which then dictates its marching orders to your DNA, cells, and proteins. Sentience is in charge of all functions when it *fully* asserts itself. Your RNA is initially programmed at the higher frequencies within your energetic templates prior to incarnating and contains the blueprint for optimum health. It's the accumulation of misprogrammed energy—the egoic identity—that throws optimum health and vitality off its tracks. But the Self can turn off what the belief-based egoic identity has miscreated.

Client Example: Lyme Disease, Anxiety, Insomnia, Hyperthyroidism

When I met Jim, he had been suffering from muscle pain, fatigue, joint pain, insomnia, and hyperthyroidism for more than ten years.

An advertising executive from Tucson and father of twin daughters, Jim had been prescribed antianxiety and thyroid medications and been diagnosed with Lyme disease. When weight lifting, yoga, herbal tinctures, a complete change in diet, acupuncture, infrared sauna, meditation, detox, and even ionized foot baths didn't result in deep or lasting improvements, a mutual friend suggested he contact me.

During our first remote session, it was obvious that Jim's thought pattern, which is how the egoic identity runs its program of limitations, was causing great disharmony. While very open-minded and a sharp reader of other people, Jim could not see his own egoic programming. Thus, every thought, feeling, action, and experience was either an affront or a validation of his sense of "self."

Jim couldn't re-create the experience of better health because an aspect of his egoic identity was misidentification with poor health and being a victim. An additional challenge was that we can't create better health and truly heal *within* if our return to health is conditional upon something outside the Self. Jim, like so many, was attached to the idea that what he needed to get better was somewhere out there—in antibiotics, tinctures, vaccines, exotic treatments, cleaner food, or whatever the latest "spiritualist" or science expert was touting. "The answer exists out there if I can only find it" is an illusion or spell. This belief, like all beliefs, is severely disempowering and therefore drains the life force instead of supporting it. As we explored this, he realized that his mindset was disempowering him and only perpetuating ill health. This was revelatory for him and maybe for you as well. In fact, the egoic identity can disguise itself as empowering by convincing you that you need to seek outside the Self even more.

As Jim and I spoke, he was able to see how *identifying* with beliefs, expectations, ruminations, ill health, thoughts, feelings, memories, and so-called knowledge were *preventing* a state of harmony. He began to see that he was making it impossible for repair and healing to germinate *within*. His egoic identity had been creating and aiding ill health while simultaneously preventing true healing.

I guided him through the very simple shortcut meditation from step 1 on letting go of baggage (on page 68) that allows pure harmonious divinity to regain dominion over the body/mind complex. When he opened his eyes, he said, "I've been meditating, or at least I always thought I had been meditating, off and on for years, but I have never had this profound sense of peace, well-being, and freedom before. Never. It's overwhelming."

"This sense of peace, well-being, and freedom is what you really are," I said. "You have been pretending to be something you can never be: flawed. Jim is just a temporary creation that was built upon many limitations. The Self is free, and now you know that experientially."

He smiled and dabbed the tears that were still flowing. "I don't ever want to lose this feeling."

"You can't," I said. "It *is* you. But when you place attention upon the egoic identity, you lose the direct connection with the Self and its innate freedom. I want you to repeat this meditation again after lunch, after dinner, and before you lie down for sleep. You need to give your body a chance to heal by unburdening itself from the stranglehold of the false self."

He promised that he would, and the next day he texted me and said he was able to sleep the entire night for the first time in years.

I shared with Jim that non-thought is how our sentience regains detachment and separation from the egoic identity and the disharmonious physical body. Now the temporary experience of both body and mind is seen with increased detachment and clarity. Any ill health our body of energy is experiencing can now be worked with properly and, if we're determined enough, transmuted back into harmony.

A few days later, we reconnected to discuss his Lyme disease diagnosis, and I shared my assessment. "Your thyroid is completely out of whack from the Lyme disease. Just as the egoic identity is a limitation program that runs by thinking, illnesses run like a program as well, which we call symptoms. They each do what they will do based upon their programming, which includes limited adapt-ability for survival."

Jim nodded. "That makes sense."

"When we perceive any physical phenomena, it's because we're perceiving the phenomenon through our temporary physical vehi-cle's senses that are attuned to the same lower frequencies as the phenomenon itself. It's why we can see our friends who are incar-nate but can no longer see the ones who have transitioned out of this range of frequencies. Understand?"

He smiled. "When you say it like that, yes."

"The blueprint of form originates or is created in much higher frequencies and dimensions," I said. "Just like building a physical structure, you have to think about its form and shape first. Form, at its origination of conception, is nothing more than structured design patterns from higher creative realms of consciousness. The higher realms affect the deeper systems within your body. If you access the chemist realm where biology is structured, you can turn off the pro-gram of illness that you are running."

"Remember that all realms are creative realms. So you're essen-tially going to turn off what no longer serves you. You can't achieve this through weak and ineffectual thoughts produced by the finite mind. You will access these higher realms through the clarity and stillness of your higher consciousness." From there, we moved on to turn off the program of illness, which you will also have the chance to do after this story.

During the meditation, Jim wept, and I knew the emotional cleans-ing was needed. By mastering step 6 over the course of roughly a month, Jim successfully turned off the program of Lyme disease and hyperthyroidism. These ill health programs had been running for nearly a decade, and now the symptoms of pain and fatigue are gone. His insomnia is gone and he sleeps restfully and consistently. Jim's energy level has increased dramatically too. He feels like his old self again, except much wiser and empowered for having healed himself. His misidentification with being ill is gone because the illness has been turned off and permanently severed. Just like your lamp when it's not plugged in, it simply doesn't work. Jim tangibly knows through his direct experience that sentient, directed intention powerfully commands energy. He is rejuvenated, has opened his own business, and has restored a quality of life that had been missing for over a decade.

Step 6 Core Exercise: Meditation to Turn Off the Program of Illness

Here is the simplest and the most expedient way to access the deeper levels of misprogramming within the energetic templates. This is precisely what I had to learn to do for myself when I experienced life-threatening autonomic dysreflexia. I accessed the deeper programs that run on automatic pilot and were misfiring because of my catastrophic spinal injury.

First, I want you to leave all delusions behind by directly tuning in to your sentience:

- Using one hand, gently place the tips of your middle and index fingers in the center of your chest.
- Bring all of your attention to that sensation of your fingers touching the center of your chest.
- Gently reach out from inside your chest and touch your fingertips.
- Feel the heart chakra open, which is the direct engagement of the Self.
- Stay there until the mind is silent and the body is perfectly still.
- Imagine in your mind's eye a digital screen that lists the programs of ill health your genetic entity is running, such as diabetes, anxiety, cancer, autoimmune disease, Lyme disease, fibromyalgia, ADHD, heart disease, hypothyroidism, etc.
- Notice that these words are illuminated like neon signs for you to recognize all the ill health programs currently running.

- Set your intention to permanently unplug any ill health programs like you would unplug a cord from an electrical outlet.
- Permanently unplug all illuminated ill health programs so they go dim.
- Now sever your electrical connections like you would cut an electrical wire. Cut them in half.
- Repeat these steps until you experience the direct tangible knowingness that you have permanently disabled and disconnected all programs of illness.
- Once you unplug and sever all ill health, *know* that it has been accomplished. You are no longer connected to nor running any programs of ill health. You have disconnected and permanently cut their energy source. This is no different than when you unplug a lamp. It is no longer connected to the energy it needs to run. Neither are the programs of ill health that the egoic identity and physical body were running. Have zero doubts that you have done this.

Because the disharmonious misprogramming of illness had garnered energetic momentum—like wearing out a patch of grass in your backyard from taking the same route over and over—the physical body and your larger, more subtle body of energy may exhibit residual symptoms of misprogramming. Give your energy field the adjustment period it needs to acclimate to its new healthy flow and path. Muscle testing will demonstrate how the physical body has responded to its ill health programs being permanently turned off and severed. Also pay attention to your dietary cravings. Desiring more natural, nutrient-dense food is a great sign that the body has begun healing itself. By turning off the program of illness, your entire body will seek different, healthier fuel to sustain its new level of health and repair.

Once you have turned off the program of illness, start to see food as information or code you feed into your biological computer—the physical body. The strongest, most robust code is that which was directly written by nature itself. These types of dietary changes will help keep any further misprogramming from entering your biological computer. For a higher-consciousness understanding of how fasting can be used to enhance self-healing, please see the appendix at the end of the book.

Step 7

Use the Power of the Spoken Word

The breath, when utilized to birth the vibration of a spoken word, greatly affects energy. Step 7 teaches you how to utilize the ancient power within the spoken word for repair, self-healing, and a greater quality of life.

Vibration, or sound, was used for therapeutic purposes throughout antiquity, and true healers have continued to use it ever since. But when scientists refused to acknowledge physical evidence that it worked, they put it in the same category as placebos. Oddly enough, the placebo effect is scientific proof that we do heal ourselves. Now, hundreds of years later, sound or vibrational therapy is becoming recognized as a highly effective tool for repair and healing of physical, emotional, mental, and energetic disharmony. Personally, I utilize direct, truthful conversations born of my higher consciousness with a myriad of clients, and their enhanced well-being is nothing short of remarkable. Today, there are all sorts of sound therapies available, but the most powerful vibration or form of sound self-therapy is still underutilized. This ultimate potency is fully realized when the vibration, or sound, being produced is closest to its source—your own truthful voice.

Prayer, mantras, invocations, and commands are highly effective because they literally reprogram the brain's current conditioning (disharmonious thought processes are the cause of all disharmony), which is how the egoic identity runs its program of limitations—by "thinking." When done masterfully, a spoken vibration that comes directly from your perfect sentience powerfully affects the entirety of your body of energy.

In order to more fully understand the power of transformation that's available through speech, think of the physical body as a structure that simply houses divinity (sentience and energy). Just as it is with the structure and function of a house, it's the empty space within it that provides the value of the structure itself. A house is essentially a hollow container meant to be filled with love, communion, joy, wisdom, happiness, and peace—a safe space or container for all that is truly divine and precious.

The same holds true for the human container. The human form was designed as an instrument to house unconditional love and timeless wisdom, and when we express our wisdom and love—our current level of self-awareness—the voice is perfectly in tune and pitch with our unique vibratory signature. The spoken word is the life energy or cosmic vibratory force of creation itself expressed through humanity's use of speech. Makes you think twice about using your voice to cast judgment, doesn't it? It destroys the energy where it originates first, my friends. It destroys the one who does the judging.

Additionally, the obvious analogy is how we manipulate each other through speech. Your spoken words are sent forth (after affecting your own energy first), which then changes the vibration within the energy field of the person you're speaking with. They get vibrationally shifted or convinced (or not convinced) due to your use of speech and its direct impact upon their energy. Great salespeople understand this and can make a comfortable living by doing it. They may not understand it from a higher-consciousness or purely energetic perspective, but they certainly comprehend how it pertains to their closing ratio and commissions.

Sounds are energy that is imbued with the life force itself and contains a specific vibration or set of vibrations. *Vibration* is another word for *information.* Vibrations affect the ether. The direct effect upon the ether that specific sounds have is how we first derived the "meaning" of sounds. This formalized way of communicating became language. Speech captures the intention of the life force and its subsequent vibrational effect upon existence. This is why prayer, mantras, invocations, and commands have been a part of the human experience since well before recorded history.

In actuality, we "spell" words because they authentically cast an energetic, vibratory effect upon existence. As mentioned previously, energy affects energy, period. Speech that is powerfully commanded by clarity, wisdom, and love creates transformation. The more sentience and focused intention that's harnessed, the more transformative and powerful its effect becomes. Your sentience has a specific and unique vibrational signature. That signature, or vibration, is the amount of love, wisdom, and power that is You.

In the beginning was the word. And that word was *sound.*

Sound shapes and creates upon the energy that is existence itself.

Generally speaking, between prayer, mantras, and spoken commands, prayer is the weakest in efficacy as it pertains to pure energetics or metaphysics. That is because prayer is often done under the assumption of separation, hierarchy, and distance. There is the person doing the praying, the entity to whom that person is praying, and finally the dispensation from that distant entity to the person who is praying or being prayed for. The belief in separation, hierarchy, and distance limits the prayer's efficacy.

Mantras are essentially the repetition of an invocation and tend to be the most effective in changing the flow of our energy patterns simply because of the repetition. But a single command spoken with complete devotion by a highly sentient and powerful being can effect the greatest transformation upon existence.

The best use of vibration, or sound, for therapeutic repair and healing is potent words associated with your sentience's preferred avenue of consciousness, which you identified in chapter 3.

As a reminder, these are the preferred avenues:

1. Reason (intellect/wisdom)
2. Faith (direct connection to your essence/totality)
3. Emotions and feelings (love)
4. Will (the life force itself, or Holy Ghost)

I used one mantra throughout my entire time in the rehabilitation hospital. Of all the avenues of consciousness, I most resonate with my will because I know that once it's fully harnessed, it cannot be stopped. Neither can yours. But in order to fully understand the power of speech, you must first fully understand your power and how it's activated. It is through the direct harnessing of the Self that transformation takes place.

The Self is sentience, the divine intelligence of the creator within us all. It is the master of all. When you say "I am," it activates the life force, the energy of creativity itself, the direct creator within you. Everything you ever undertake, be it thought or action, starts with "I am." Ultimately, what you really are is limitless, divine, and utterly complete, so that anything you place after "I am" is not you but rather the experience you are creating.

I am going to work. I am going to get something to eat. I am going to think about that. I am feeling good about that. I am wondering. "I am" is the Self, or sentience, engaged. It harnesses your body of energy into creator mode by command. Whatever you choose to place after "I am" creates and dictates your experience in this life and every other.

The command I employed repetitively as a mantra was simply this:

I am the conqueror of my mind and body.

This mantra, when said with total conviction and devotion, will empower you beyond any mental or emotional comprehension. I used this mantra, and only this mantra, as a multiplier of my kinetic intention to put my paralyzed and ravaged body back together—to supercharge the reconstruction of my body of energy. If this one doesn't feel right to you, you can create your own. We'll look at this more in the core exercise for this chapter.

Client Example: Stage 4 Breast Cancer

When Leslie was diagnosed with stage 4 breast cancer, her partner, a real estate developer, knew the battle she had ahead of her and suggested that she meet with me to see if I felt whether anything could be done to slow or reverse her condition. He was very concerned and desperately wanted her to get help.

Two days later, I met with Leslie in my office. She told me that her doctors were very pessimistic. "They say my chance of survival is not encouraging."

I knew the perils of identifying with a diagnosis, but I wanted her to come to that conclusion herself, so I said, "How do you feel about that?"

She shook her head. "I don't agree. I'm going to heal myself. That's why I came here today."

We were off to a great start. I said, "Your opinion is the only one that matters when it comes to your healing. When you refuse to accept and love yourself, even in the face of great adversity, disharmony brews. If you simmer that festering concoction long enough, it boils over and spreads. It eventually takes on a life of its own."

Leslie removed her glasses and rubbed the bridge of her nose. She was hurting, but she summoned the will to ask, "Do you think it's treatable, or is it already too late?"

"What do you think?"

She sat up straighter, broadening her shoulders. "I know I can heal myself. Whatever it takes, I'm determined to do it."

I smiled. "That's all that matters. Let's get to work."

She nodded in agreement and smiled.

"What is paramount, Leslie, is your state of being. Your complete intention must be directed upon healing yourself. You must remove all doubt. Are you ready to do that?"

"Absolutely. Will you show me what I need to do, specifically?"

"Of course. But first you must *know*, not believe, that you will heal yourself."

"I understand."

I explained that she was going to command her own healing by harnessing the life force through the spoken word. I explained how specific sounds affect energy in specific ways (as mentioned earlier). When repeated with the utmost fervor, devotion, and conviction, mantras have a powerful effect on the body of energy subjected to their intention. The more powerfully you perform the mantras, the larger the body of energy you affect, and with greater efficacy. Mantras can literally change the program of illness on the deepest levels. It's why people do affirmations. It rewires their brain, which in turn redirects the energy flow within the body. Through repeated command, mantras pause the current misprogramming. They then enhance the electrical intention of the intelligent consciousness within our body of energy for its self-repair and self-healing design. I asked Leslie which of the four directions of healing resonated most with her: reason, faith, emotions and feelings, or will.

Without batting an eye, Leslie said, "Faith."

So I shared this mantra with her:

> *God is within me, and I am with God.*
> *My body is healed by thy lightning rod.*

It immediately resonated with Leslie.

I said, "I want you to calm yourself. Breathe deeply from your diaphragm until the mind and body are still. Really connect with the words; don't just say them. Now, with sincere devotion and fervor, speak from the depths of your soul and recognize the truth. Do it now."

As she repeated her mantra, tears streamed down her cheeks. I logged in to her energy field. Her true faith was being expressed powerfully and sincerely. Her devotion and connection to the words was changing her energy. By sincerely saying the word *God*, her attention was upon God, and so she was connecting with that energy directly. Color was returning to her gray complexion.

"Do this mantra as much as you can," I said. "Marry yourself to the vibration it creates within you. Fill yourself with Light so nothing impure can remain."

Leslie was resolute and promised she would continue to do it, as well as schedule sessions with me moving forward. She left my office completely resolute in her knowingness that she would heal herself through her mantras.

At each of our scheduled follow-up sessions, I logged in to her, and each time the cancer had shrunk since the last visit. The color in her face was much better, and the swelling in her neck had almost disappeared.

Leslie said that her mantra was creating a huge ball of white light that encompassed the cancer and kept shrinking it and shrinking it. She was absolutely right. At the end of the month, her doctor informed her that the mass had shrunk dramatically. She said her medical team could not understand or explain how this was possible. Because of the huge reduction in both masses, Leslie saw no harm in having radiation treatments, which she had already paid for anyway. Her situation was now deemed treatable by Western medicine. After the rounds of radiation, Leslie informed me that the doctors told her there was no mass in one specific location, and just an empty cavity in the other location where cancer had been previously. Remarkably, Leslie was cancer-free.

The complete mastery of mantras gives us the power to create transformation and healing well beyond what is perceivable to the five physical senses. Leslie healed herself because of her mastery of step 7 of the ATFHT. Her complete faith, devotion, and alignment with the healing vibration of her very own words saved her physical life. Such is the power at the disposal of each and every person.

Step 7 Core Exercise: Mantras for Healing through the Spoken Word

You can use one of the mantras below that's aligned with your preferred avenue of healing, or you can create one yourself. Always have mantras come from the Self, your truth, and not your egoic identity. Do not reach for a mantra, but rather discover it deep within yourself. What resonates most deeply within the Self will come forward if you keep your attention there. Do not allow the finite mind to censor your truth. The finite mind is a parasite and tangibly knows nothing.

If you are creating your own mantra, choose the words wisely. Keep your mantras (commands) in the present tense, simple and direct. If your mantra is not in the present tense, your manifestation cannot occur now. Repeat them out loud with fervor and sincere devotion, and they will rewire your disharmonious thought process and repair your larger body of energy. Do the mantra you choose as much as you can. Marry yourself to the vibration it creates within you. Say it out loud.

Below is a mantra for each avenue of consciousness.

Now calm yourself. Breathe deeply from your diaphragm until the mind and body are still. Really connect with the words; don't just say them. With sincere devotion and fervor, speak from your soul and recognize the truth. Do it now.

Will Mantra
I am the conqueror of my mind and body.
My power commands all that is godly.

Emotion Mantra
I am love, I am joy.
All disharmony I destroy.

Faith Mantra

God is within me, and I am with God.
My body is healed, thy holiest sod.

Reason Mantra

I am the design of perfect health.
My healing power is the truest wealth.

Do not be surprised if you experience overwhelming emotional states, an immense activation of power, or a heightened state of clarity and consciousness as a result of these mantras. When performed with the surrender of complete conviction of the Total Self, they harness the power of transformation itself.

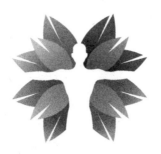

Conclusion

Maintain Your New Pattern of Harmony through Continued Practice

What you have done in order to manifest your repair and healing is the reawakening of the Self. This new perspective born of self-awareness, which you utilized to command healing in previous steps, leads to a better quality of life. Your awakened Self is the key to maintaining an optimum state of perpetual vitality, health, and well-being. Moving forward, your continued practice of the steps will keep you in this positive state.

Healing Comes in Many Forms

When we see or hear the word *healing*, we tend to think of physical healing because it's the most obvious form from the perspective of our limited sensory perceptions. The real reason physical healing comes to mind first is because the egoic identity automatically identifies itself with the body. This misidentification happens instantaneously, and without self-awareness we don't understand what and why it really occurred. Without true self-awareness, we imprison ourselves within the limitations of body consciousness and the fragmentations born of misperceptions, misunderstandings, and misidentifications we call thoughts. The result is always wanting or craving something, and that state of being is a poor quality of life.

Sometimes we heal emotionally or mentally from an experience, but we remain injured physically. Sometimes we heal physically but remain mentally or emotionally traumatized. There are also cases where the physical body or finite mind is not directly harmed, but the larger body of energies becomes traumatized indirectly from misidentifying with something that it deems sufficiently unpleasant. There are innumerable combinations of the various depths of misidentifications within all of these elements, both individually and collectively. The one thing they all have in common is a lack of self-awareness. Suffering is inevitable when identification is created. The Self does not and cannot suffer, ever. It simply observes in acceptance. The egoic identity and its misprogrammed body of energy is what suffers.

As with any challenge, including health, when you do your absolute best, moment to moment, regardless of the outcome, you are evolving at your maximum rate and capacity. This is the highest use of all experience. Always doing your best also provides inspiration for others to do the same.

It's not the duration of our temporary incarnation that matters, but the quality, depth, and richness of our experience of Self in relation to the outer world. In other words, being fully present is the key. True consciousness evolution is the accrual of sentience, and it is occurring with the greatest efficacy when experientially we know what, why, and how our challenges have arisen and to work with these experiences to the absolute best of our ability. This is how we accrue sentience—how we deepen our reservoir of love, wisdom, and power. This occurs when the Self is leading the incarnation. The Self is fully online only in the unencumbered, unfiltered, and unlimited now.

In terms of repair and overall health, some souls signed up for spontaneous healing, fast healing, gradual healing, slow healing, or no healing. This is within the life plan itself. This also applies to all the different forms of healing, (mental, emotional, physical, energetic). The Self is already perfect and immortal. It's always creatively engaged in play. It's how we accept and work with our planned challenges that dictate the quality of life and the efficacy of our evolution. The only true measure of success is personal happiness. Move through this realm in freedom and joy.

Sentience cannot get sick or die, but the physical body must eventually, even for those who have achieved transformation through authentic self-mastery. What has a beginning always has an ending. Know, beyond a shadow of a doubt, that you are much more than what comes and goes. Discover your Self by practicing the ATFHT. We can all work with our challenges in a more advanced, holistic fashion and discover the infinite possibilities we all inherently have to transform and transcend our current state of being. We are all capable and destined to improve our health, quality of life, depth of sentience, and functionality. Do not identify the Self with the current human form or its agreed-upon limitations. Both of these temporary placeholders have yet to be fully transmuted by your awakened, immortal creator Self.

We never actually own anything, including sickness or health. They are simply temporary, reflective experiences.

You—the Self—are a fractal of divinity, freedom, and perfection. The Total Self is your love, wisdom, and complement of energy. You do not take the physical body, identity, brain, knowledge, stuff, friends, family, pets, money, cars, jewelry, job title, or anything with you when your body perishes. It's amazing how we spend our entire lifetime perpetuating, hoarding, and protecting all that does not endure. It's pointless, and you deserve better in every way.

You are eternally and infinitely more than the finite mind and temporary body can ever contain or express.

You Are No Longer a Master of Limitations but Rather a Limitless Master

Continue to be the embodiment of graceful and fearless determination. The Self is the ultimate treasure and your greatest discovery. You have triumphed over your suffering and ill health. Don't look back or reach for the old identity and its programmed misbehaviors and habits of disharmony. Your new state of being and the empowering, harmonious expressions you have manifested must be maintained with gentle, unwavering tenacity.

"I feel better now, so I can go back to what I used to do" is a trick of the egoic identity to regain control and dominion over your imagination, freedom, and body of energy. Don't take the bait. If you do, it will cause a new version of your previous ill health programming by essentially reliving the disharmonious thoughts, emotions, actions, and behaviors of the egoic identity. The past, your false self, will recreate its previous reality that can never serve your highest potential.

When you grab hold of a thought, bring it closer, and ruminate on it, you lose all freedom and clarity. All you can experience is the thought itself. There is no freedom or harmony in thinking. Through repetition of the exercises in step 1, you'll discover an ancient secret: All thoughts are empty and equal in weightlessness. It's simply your indulgence and belief in a thought that gives it its weight and sway over your freedom, clarity, and body of energy. Don't think; *know*. Trust the Self.

The same goes for feelings, experiences, and knowledge. Existence itself is a blank canvas, an empty container, and either you fill it with your misperceptions, misunderstandings, and misidentifications or you create from the unlimited and never-ending imagination that is your higher consciousness.

You are a powerful Creator. The "what" you are trying to achieve and the "who" that performs the actions are merely temporary energetic placeholders, creations of your own imagination. Make sure these temporary placeholders are worthy of your true divinity, freedom, perfection, and limitless imagination.

The Self wants to perpetually unfurl and expand in order to experientially know itself. The only obstacles that prevent this continuous expansion are what we place in the way; namely, the limitations we self-impose through misperceptions, misunderstandings, and misidentifications. *Thinking*. All thinking is always in context to a belief.

So-called knowledge, authority, concepts, fears, beliefs, memories, and prejudice only hold the limitless Self in bondage. Whatever you hold on to becomes your prison and warden. Don't hold on to anything, and nothing will have a hold over you.

For hundreds, maybe even thousands, of years, the running of a sub-four-minute mile was deemed absolutely and unequivocally humanly impossible. It was an accepted fact that it was simply beyond what the human body could ever do. Then, in 1954, a British elite runner named Roger Bannister finally broke that illusory barrier. He achieved the impossible. Once he did, it gave everyone permission to do the same. Six weeks later, someone else did it. All of a sudden, others began to break that once impossible barrier too. Once it is downloaded into the collective consciousness, it suddenly becomes possible for all.

Summary of the Ascend the Frequencies Healing Technique

The ATFHT is now within the collective consciousness. It is a permission slip for you to do the impossible for yourself. As a reminder, here is a summary of the entire process.

Before diving into the steps of the ATFHT, figure out how to utilize the four directions of consciousness for self-healing, which are (1) reason, (2) emotions and feelings, (3) faith, and (4) will. Through the protocols in chapter 3, you are able to determine which or what combination of these avenues works best for you. Just as it's exhausting and ultimately pointless to resist the current of a river, let your life force flow in complete accordance with your chosen direction. This is the opposite of effort. Once the preferred method(s) is determined, you can surrender to the eternal flow of your own life force. From there, we move along to the steps of the program.

Step 1: Access Your True Essence

Summary: Let go of your ego/mind/identity (EMI) and access your true essence.

Purpose: These simple yet immensely powerful and transformative protocols dissolve the illusion of the ego/mind/identity, which is the cause of all suffering and ill health. The core exercises help you to connect with your true essence.

Practice:

- Shortcuts to Dissolve the Ego/Mind/Identity
  - —Ask Yourself, "Who Am I?"
  - —Let Go of Baggage (Past, Future, and Thought)
  - —Fingers to Chest
  - —Imagine You're a Pair of Eyes Floating in Space
  - —Say "I Don't Know"
  - —Clear Old Disharmonious Thought Patterns
  - —Clear Old Disharmonious Emotional Patterns
- Meditations to Log In to Your True Essence
  - —Part 1: Feeling Your True Essence through Observation
  - —Part 2: Logging In to Assess Your Energy

Frequency of Use: Perform all steps as needed until the egoic identity no longer has control over your consciousness and its body of energy. Being the Self (the unblocked parasympathetic and transformational state) will be your new habit. All healing potential and quality of life resides here.

Step 2: Know Specifically What You Are Going to Achieve

Summary: Separate from your doubts and know specifically what you are going to achieve. Ask yourself the question "What specifically do I want to achieve?" Refine your answer multiple times through repeat questioning, and once complete, clearly and definitively write down the final statement. The more fine-tuned and specific your answer, the more power you can bring to its fruition.

Purpose: Rather than doubting, you can marry yourself to the vibration of victory already within you. This step will help you learn how to never waver in your conviction, so that the tangible recognition of your intention and desire must manifest. Once the desired achievement is written, the energetic contract is always in force, unless you willfully break it.

Practice:

- Shortcuts to Separate Yourself from Your Doubts
    - —Countering Doubt Pop-Ins
    - —Unfollow Your Doubts
- Set Your Intention and Desire

Frequency of Use: Every morning and every evening, reestablish and realign your specific intention. This will free up your neural pathways from limitation programming and unleash your energetic power to manifest your intention.

Step 3: Activate Your Healing Intention

Summary: Activate the state of healing with the intention you created in step 2. See (imagine), feel, perform, and verbalize your action. As you're seeing/feeling/doing this, acknowledge that you are commanding your vital energy by utilizing the breath of life. Say out loud, "I repair and heal my (blank) now. With every movement, my (blank) is energized, repaired, made whole."

Purpose: This step utilizes all fundamental human expression (mental, emotional, physical, and verbal) and activates the intention/desire. This step can be thought of this way: mental visualization + physical action + emotional stimulation + the spoken word = activation of your healing intention.

Practice:

- Mental Visualization
- Physical Action
- Emotional Stimulation
- Spoken Word

Frequency of Use: Daily, in the same way you would approach your exercise regimen or your yoga or meditation practice. Thirty to sixty minutes total broken into intervals or sets is optimal.

Step 4: Command Creator Consciousness

Summary: Learn how to access these higher states of consciousness. This step provides the ultimate high-frequency meditation where you can access the higher realm of the universal, omniscient, and omnipotent higher mind of Source. Follow the meditation instructions faithfully. Record yourself and/or have someone guide you, then you guide them.

Purpose: Higher consciousness is the chemist of our biology and the architect of our form. Accessing and commanding this high-frequency energy helps to repair and heal at the root and not just treat symptoms. Like an Etch A Sketch, access your higher consciousness and re-create yourself.

Practice:

• Healing Meditation to Command Creator Consciousness

Frequency of Use: Repeat this meditation daily. Feel free to do it multiple times a day.

Step 5: Channel Intelligent Energy into the Body

Summary: Access Intelligent Energy by channeling it into your body through the crown chakra. Imagine a never-ending waterfall of healing energy cascading down through the top of head and filling your body. Follow the instructions in order to open your crown chakra and command or download Intelligent Energy into and through your body of energy. You can also have the Intelligent Energy pour out your mini palm chakras and/or heart chakra and onto whatever body part, organ, or system needs repair.

Purpose: Access Intelligent Energy, which has the innate ability to transmute lower frequency disharmony, in order to repair and heal yourself.

Practice:

- Channel Intelligent Energy through the Crown Chakra

Frequency of Use: Bring Intelligent Energy into and through your area of disharmony and sickness as often as you like, but not less than once a day. Multiple sessions of twenty minutes per session provide ample opportunity for Intelligent Energy's innate ability to transmute lower frequency disharmony.

Step 6: Turn Off the Program of Illness

Summary: Turn off, unplug, and sever the connections to illness (like you would unplug and take down a neon sign). By accessing the higher frequencies, where the building blocks of our form and function exist, we learn to apply step 6 to literally turn off the program of illness we are running.

Purpose: Symptoms are simply the tangible subset of various programs of limitation that we acquire and run called illness and disease. Like all programs, they were added and therefore can be turned off and deleted. Your mind/body complex (biological computer) runs best with the least number of programs running on its hard drive. It is no different than turning off a light and unplugging it from its power source: once done, the light is permanently off. The same is true when we turn off and delete the program of illness we are running. The illness no longer has an energy source to sustain itself.

Practice:

- Meditation to Turn Off the Program of Illness

Frequency of Use: Once daily is sufficient, or twice a day, once upon waking and again before bed.

Step 7: Use the Power of the Spoken Word

Summary: Utilize the ancient power within the spoken word for repair, self-healing, and a greater quality of life. Reharmonize your entire body of energy through commands, mantras, and affirmations. Let your Self's supremely high vibration regain total dominion over your incarnation by verbalizing your divinity, perfection, freedom, and victory.

Purpose: Vibration, or sound, has been used for therapeutic purposes throughout antiquity, and true healers have continued to use it ever since. Our most powerful vibration is the internal dialogue we speak directly from the Self to our conscious mind and body of energy. Lower frequency disharmony cannot exist within a supremely high-vibrational environment. As Buddha is believed to have said, "What we think, we become. What we imagine, we create. What we feel, we attract." Expression through speech can ensure your complete victory and liberation from disharmony.

Practice:

- Mantras for Healing through the Spoken Word

Frequency of Use: Repeat your commands and mantras multiple times daily until your entire body of energy resonates in complete union with them.

Once we've found harmony through the practice of these steps, the goal is to maintain this new pattern. Live the new understandings and repeat the intention, thoughts, emotions, actions, and behaviors born directly from the Self that fostered your better health and quality of life. The Self that broke the habits of disharmony is now online, and we need to avoid the return to old habits. Live as the rediscovered Self, and the limitations of your egoic identity (which includes misidentification with illness) shall no longer be your reality. As the false self dissolves, so does its story of ill health and poor quality of life. Never look back or forward. Simply do what you tangibly know to be true and expect no results. This is perpetual harmony.

Remember, utilize the new understandings and tangible experience of the protocols within step 1 to reclaim your freedom and life force and to effortlessly maintain the "no mind" state. The empty mind/calm state is the starting point for true transformation.

If you're not seeing results, it's because you're not supposed to be looking for them. Stay within the process of creating. Seeking results is attaching yourself to a possible future outcome based upon your perceived past. Rather than seeking, empty your mind and calm your emotions. How? Simply pretend that you just arrived here, with no past and no future. Now there is no story you keep projecting about your health and state of being. This gives you back the freedom and harmony you always had. Now you can powerfully create.

Dedicate yourself completely to the new understandings and exercises and tangibly see for yourself. Experience what is truly possible for an ultimate creator being. The ATFHT was born of the wisdom that transcends knowledge. Use it with the utmost fervor and sincerity imbued by your faithfulness, love, and devotion. Use it, my friends, like the Master you already are!

The keys to greater well-being, personal growth, repair, self-healing, and liberation exist within the Self, not within your finite mind or body consciousness. The ATFHT gives you—the explorer—the treasure map for the greatest hero's journey you will ever take: the journey of Self-mastery. The work you do now by accessing and commanding your Total Self not only directly impacts the quality of this life but also pays you eternal dividends in every simultaneous, parallel, and concurrent condition.

Commit to each step of the ATFHT and a greater quality of life, repair, and health will manifest. It will not be a coincidence, because coincidences don't actually exist. What exists are immutable and eternal laws captured within the steps of this practice that make self-healing our destiny.

What is possible through sincere devotion and disciplined adherence to all the steps of the ATFHT is boundless, because it taps into the limitless nature of your higher consciousness. There are no limitations on what can be achieved when you access what is truly unlimited. Not only have I seen firsthand my own impossible transcendence but I have seen others do it themselves as well. Now it's your turn.

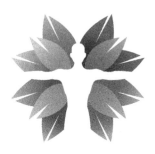

Appendix

Fasting as It Relates to Turning Off the Program of Illness

What does fasting accomplish in terms of repair and self-healing from a heightened consciousness perspective?

There is a copious amount of great scientific data that backs up the incredible efficacy of fasting in regard to anti-aging as well as the repair and healing of sickness and disease. So many wonderful studies illustrate what medically supervised fasting can do, and I strongly encourage you to avail yourself of this proven method. My interest in fasting as it relates to turning off the program of illness is to provide a higher-consciousness understanding that isn't discoverable through the physical senses or intellect.

As we learned earlier, the key to achievement of any goal is to ask yourself, "What specifically am I trying to achieve?" The more specific we are, the more we harness our energy with single-pointedness of concentration, which powerfully unleashes our full creative potential.

Here are some of the goals we may have in mind when considering fasting:

- Weight loss
- Fat burning
- Growth hormone release

- Anti-aging
- Detox
- Self-control (eliminate unhealthy eating habits)
- Self-discipline (learning new healthy habits)
- Autophagy (meaning "self-devouring"—the natural, regulated mechanism of the cell that removes unnecessary and dysfunctional components)
- Self-healing
- Self-awareness

The following is a higher consciousness perspective regarding a twenty-one-day fast that I conducted on myself.

Let's begin with the analogy of a sleek, sophisticated submarine and how it functions properly, as opposed to the disharmonious egoic identity and its disastrous effect upon our body of energy including the human vehicle. A submarine does all of its work and serves its purpose when it is submerged in the ocean, sometimes miles deep. Because of its elegant and superior design, a submarine runs smoothly and perfectly even in the harshest of environments. The moment it takes anything in from its massive work environment—water—it immediately begins to falter, systems malfunction, critical performance breaks down, and it eventually sinks.

The human vessel works exactly the same way. It was designed to perfection for the purpose and experience of the immortal Self for incarnation within the lower frequencies of the physical universe. Our body of energy, which includes the animation of the human vehicle, runs perfectly and smoothly when it ceases to take in anything (in-formation) from its low-frequency work environment.

The accumulation of sensory-perceived information that we misidentify our Self with creates the disharmonious egoic identity. These misperceptions lead to misunderstandings, which create misidentifications. We then suffer our own creation: the ego/mind/identity (EMI) and its program of limitations. Remember, our incarnations are but tendrils extended from our Higher Self/Totality for its evolution and ascension "up" the multiverse. The Higher-Self/Totality needs the physical vehicle for its projected Total Self—you—to experience this low frequency. Your complement of energy is of a supremely high frequency. By misidentifying the Self with anything of this realm, you attach your harmonious, high-frequency body of energy to a low frequency. This causes great mental, emotional, physical, and energetic distress.

Like the submarine, the human vehicle or vessel runs smoothly, efficiently, and optimally when it takes in *nothing* from its local environment.

This applies to all "information," whether in the form of beliefs/non-beliefs/so-called knowledge and even, to a staggering degree, what we call *food*. Yes, even food. *Information* is another word for *vibration*, and when we "take in" any information, it alters the harmonious functionality and self-repair/self-healing program that our vessel is designed for. If we already have a supercomputer but we keep downloading more and more programs onto its hard drive, this will minimize its previous efficiency, self-cleaning, and self-regulating internal mechanisms and its functional performance. The body/mind complex works exactly the same way.

Humanity is currently under the influence of a myriad of misperceptions regarding the physical vehicle or vessel. It will naturally repair and heal itself if we simply cease adding constant additional rogue programmed information—in this instance, what we call food—that it must process in order to be balanced. Our normal state, believe it or not, is a perfect, self-correcting balance. From a standard consciousness perspective, if you firmly believe you are the body and not the sentience temporarily merged with it, then you must eat. Your beliefs make it real, and fasting would be dangerous for you. Conversely, if you tangibly know you are not the physical body but actually the sentience temporarily merged with it, you will need to eat much less in comparison, and some will need to eat only sporadically, rarely, and sometimes almost never.

We have all heard that the body is somewhere around 60 percent water. My direct understanding is that the body is mostly bacteria, electrolytes, minerals, proteins, and fats—not water. Constant hydration actually depletes the body of essential electrolytes and minerals through urination. This sends signals to the mind that the body is depleted and needs fuel/energy. We reactively consume food, which actually taxes the body in order to metabolize the food into energy.

Optimally, we would catabolize the damaged cells and proteins for energy (autophagy), which our body is designed to do if we let it. But instead, we eat food. Health, as it stands currently, is a collection of misunderstood justified beliefs that perpetuates a cycle of imbalance and ill health in order to sell various "goods" and "services" to you. This dysfunction only leads to further seeking outside of the self to fix what is designed to perfection and programmed to self-repair and self-heal. The belief-based egoic identity is the misprogramming. Due to its misidentification with the physical body, we keep feeding ourselves more "food" information instead of letting the body run properly and naturally repair and heal itself.

Remember, our chakras are energy transformers that keep our body intact and running.

Health care and the food industry are businesses—that's all—and authentic healing kills repeat business. It is not a coincidence that the mystics, yogis, shamans, and Masters throughout antiquity have performed and advocated extended fasting and meditation for repair and healing of the body for longer than recorded human history has been kept. When we see food as simply rogue information that doesn't need to be processed by a perfect biological computer that already runs its own self-repair and self-healing program, we will learn to eat far, far less, and be much healthier and happier for it. Neither food nor water is the answer to health or vitality. Health is already contained within and is our natural state. Additional information only slows down and severely throws off what is already the perfection of design and functionality born of higher consciousness.

What the "body" metabolizes is energy, but the finite lower mind, due to its deep misidentification with the physical body, "thinks" it gets it from food. From a higher consciousness perspective, we can observe our chakra system and tangibly experience that it is the energy transformer and translator that metabolizes the energies within our local frequential environment that sustains us. It is our chakras that keep our physical form intact and nourish our body of energy. A higher state of self-awareness and more expansive consciousness reveals what the physical senses and the intellect can never and will never comprehend.

The seeming necessity of constantly consuming physical food is based upon our vibration, or more specifically, the quality and quantity of sentience. This incorporates the individual's consciousness or brain wave frequency. Our depth of misidentification with the physical body and sensory phenomena (thoughts, emotions, actions) greatly determines this frequential brain wave pattern. The more we misidentify the Self with anything of low frequency (contraction of awareness), the more narrow, closed-minded, and nonaccepting we become. This way of being is akin to a beta wave state or a lower consciousness perspective. For these people, prolonged fasting could be lethal. The more self-aware (expansion of awareness) we are, the more open-minded and self-accepting we become. This creates a more expansive perspective, which is more akin to a delta wave state of higher consciousness. These are the people who would benefit a great deal from responsible, monitored fasting.

From birth to roughly seven years old, our own sentience determines how immersed its incarnation will be based upon its misidentification with the physical world, including the body. It's a determination each Self makes as the incarnation is unfolding. We can choose to be fully immersed (which translates to the experience of firmly believing that we are merely human, that we are the body/thoughts/feelings/experiences and that's it) or essentially the opposite (which translates to tangibly knowing we are sentience merely having a temporary human experience), and every limitless gradient between these two extremes. This choice that we all make greatly affects our ability to practice prolonged fasting for repair, healing, consciousness exploration, and increased vitality.

Everyone's Higher Self/Totality understands the above, but the egoic mind prevents access to the clarity of higher consciousness where the blueprint for repair and self-healing exists. Repair, healing, and vitality are paved by greater self-awareness, and it is simply our harnessing of the will, through self-control and self-discipline, that makes it happen. Self-realization means to tangibly realize the Self and where it originates from. All obfuscations have been removed. What remains is simply the complete commanding of the will to do whatever is needed to engender repair, health, and perpetual harmony.

Higher consciousness is the chemist of our biology and the architect of our form. This is what is meant by the saying that humanity is created in God's image. By accessing our higher consciousness within the universal omniscient mind of God/Source/Creator, we can greatly direct our repair and healing. The egoic identity, which acts like a spell, a limitation program, sees, treats, and understands symptoms only within the frequential range of sensory perceptions, which has nothing to do with actual healing. This is why we forever swing ourselves on the pendulum of good and poor health. Our health needs to be permanent, and these new understandings are a bridge to that inner equilibrium. We cannot learn what we think we already know, and this is true in regard to self-repair and self-healing.

Fat

Fat is burned during sleep and is dictated by the liver. Our liver has a very high degree of consciousness and is constantly at odds with the finite mind. The liver knows what to do, inherently, as do all of our organs, but the low-frequency finite mind does not. That's why the mind constantly wants more and more information—because it knows nothing. Therein lies the problem we perpetually create for our liver. It, along with our other organs, no longer trusts our finite mind, and for good reason.

Fat burning is simply a function of caloric expenditure versus intake. Fat loss (not the same as fat burning) occurs when in a parasympathetic state or more relaxed state. This is essential to understand from a higher consciousness perspective. The relaxed or parasympathetic state relates to higher brain waves or a more expanded state of consciousness. This is achieved as sentience gains dominion over the egoic mind and our body of energy. For most of us, unfortunately, it is experienced only when the false self is unconscious (sleep).

It is not a coincidence that all major fat loss, repair, and healing occurs during sleep. That is because during sleep the body/mind complex is not held hostage by the disharmonious egoic identity. We exist and operate in our natural state of higher consciousness when asleep, and it's why we don't remember anything. It would give the game away of merely being human. Remembering everything from "sleep" would reveal immediately what we have come here to consciously learn through the tangible experience of our intentions. Because we are part of this evolutionary cycle, we must heal ourselves where the misperception occurred—while incarnate and "in-time." Why? Because the bigger the challenge, the greater the triumph. This is the accrual or deepening of sentience.

The egoic identity is a lower reactionary (stress) state of consciousness. This is due to our low-frequency local environment that our body and its physical sensory perceptions are attuned to. The more we misidentify and react, the greater imbalances and ill health we create. A low-frequency existence results in a poor quality of life, whether we are "materially" successful (belief system) or not. The counter to misidentification is observation. This is why we always hear the phrases "just observe" and "be the witness." By identifying and reacting, which is the opposite of observing and responding, we cause a tsunami of disharmonious energy waves throughout our "body" of energy. This is easily identifiable with the release of stress hormones such as cortisol into the blood stream. This release of stress hormones causes a chain reaction that can express itself as anxiety, which typically leads to sleep deprivation. This state keeps your consciousness outside of the parasympathetic state needed for vitality, repair, rejuvenation, and health. This is just one example of the cause—misidentification and reaction— with the effects being disharmony and disease. The egoic mind—a lower consciousness, belief-based, non-self-aware reactionary state— also makes your blood more insulin-resistant, and therefore the body becomes increasingly toxic and unhealthy. Processing food "information" is not the answer to this problem.

Growth Hormone

Growth hormone (GH) is a peptide hormone that stimulates growth, cell reproduction, and regeneration. It has been touted for its anti-aging properties, as well as its ability to stimulate muscle growth, bone density, and fat loss. GH is released during the sleep state—non-reactionary—which is what accounts for fat burning, physical repair, and regeneration. Higher states of consciousness activate these things on their own, which simultaneously detaches one from the lower frequencies and thus misidentification with the "physical" self. The more we detach from identification with the lower frequencies, the more prominent the higher consciousness is within our waking conscious mind; this promotes the release of GH.

The beta brain wave inhibits GH release, which speeds up the aging process. This misidentification with body consciousness makes it impossible to fast. It would be seriously dangerous and possibly deadly for those with the misperceptions, misunderstandings, and misidentifications with their temporary experience of physicality. The corrosive trifecta of misperceptions, misunderstandings, and misidentifications puts constant and unrelenting stress on our body of energy, which disables its innate directive for self-repair and self-healing. Our sentience is of a monumentally higher frequency that turbo-boosts the body's natural ability for self-healing when it has regained dominion over the incarnation. The conscious return to our naturally higher state of awareness is essential for GH release, vitality, anti-aging, and health.

Hormones Are Habits

As we now understand, the belief-based egoic identity is a limitation program that runs by thinking, and the main habit of humanity is thinking. On many levels, the false self is simply a collection of habits, and it is our habits that dictate hormones. We get hungry at a certain time because we are used to eating at that time. We crave salty or sweet snacks because we have created that habit, and our hormones simply follow the directional momentum we have given them. Fasting gives the Self dominion and control over the mind/body complex on much deeper levels than we understand. Once we have broken the habit of eating, we have begun to break some of the foundational habits that make up the belief-based mental/emotional/behavioral patterns of the disharmonious egoic identity. That energy can now be used for repair and healing instead of fueling the low-frequency habits that created disharmony. Break your habits, and your hormones will behave completely differently. Then your hormones will serve your vitality and health rather than lead you astray into poor health and a lack of vitality.

Self-Control

As stated earlier, the order of creation is desire, intention, thought, emotion, action, and then behavior. Far too often, it's our reactions (programming) that fuel our creations such as thought, emotions, actions, and behaviors. Self-control is the ability to transcend reactionary impulses. The reason many of us suffer from a lack of self-control is because we have not investigated its root. No self-control is the egoic identity program of limitations simply reacting to sensory stimuli as opposed to what you really are—the Self—which chooses whether or not to respond. That is the difference between no self-control and ultimate self-control. Think of it this way: A child has not developed any control over what they say and do. They throw temper tantrums and say whatever comes to mind. If we have not learned to control our mind, emotions, and actions, then have we actually grown up or simply grown old?

When we understand the motivation behind our every desire, intention, thought, emotion, action, and behavior, we will gain supreme self-control. Our power to transcend things like poor eating habits or even just the amount of food we consume will no longer be problematic. Essentially, the who that thinks and feels the craving for rogue information to enter their body of energy to process will be gone and will no longer have sway over the freedom of ultimate self-control. Fasting for seventy-two hours reunites the conscious mind with its ability to transcend hormonal cravings and behavioral patterns. That is the starting point for gaining true self-control over poor eating. If you can fast for seventy-two hours, you can do anything. The rest is deciding what specifically you desire to achieve.

Self-control leads to self-discipline, which unlocks your power of transformation…self-mastery.

Once the power of self-control is tangibly felt, stoke this flame by feeding it your constant attention. Tangibly feel the power of your will by continuing to exercise it. One way is to just keep fasting, if you can, as long as you are under medical supervision and monitoring yourself diligently. During a prolonged fast, I would obsessively measure my blood sugar and ketone level every three hours while limiting my physical exertion. I drank plenty of electrolytes and minerals in my two liters of daily water intake. I would "log in" to myself continually throughout the day using my higher intuitive functions so I could better understand what was happening to my body of energy on very deep and subtle levels. You must be extremely aware and gentle with yourself while fasting. If you are not fully committed to paying extra loving attention to your health while having professional medical guidance during your fast, then don't do it. If you don't feel well or get light-headed, immediately drink some juice and eat.

Once you have regained great self-control through your fast, it's imperative that you maintain this power moving forward. Now is a great time to begin a true program of meditation, yoga, and exercise. Devote yourself to something that speaks directly to your heart and that will not strain your newfound self-control and self-discipline over poor eating choices or even eating much at all. The choice to fast must be done thoughtfully, always under a health practitioner's supervision, and with constant, vigilant self-monitoring and self-love. No exceptions, my friends.

Once you have repeated the use of self-control for about three weeks, you will have developed completely new pathways for your energy. The old, unhealthy pathways will have been paved over by a new, healthier way. You will have achieved a permanent neuroplasticity in your eating habits, and you will have done it the only way that is authentic—by developing your own self-control and self-discipline. These changes are ones that will last, because they were directed by the Self and now run deep within your body of energy. You will find out how little you need to eat and what best to eat to feel great, be energetic, and be healthy. Rogue programs of information that run on our biological computer, which we call illness and disease, need energy to sustain themselves. Prolonged fasting, when done properly with supervision, is one way to deprive the disharmonious programs of the electricity they need to power themselves. At the risk of sounding dogmatic and annoyingly redundant, fasting is never to be taken lightly or done without medical supervision. Never do it as a "healthy" way of being aggressive with yourself.

Autophagy

Autophagy means "self-eating" and is the body's way of removing damaged cells and proteins and replacing them with new ones. There are over a dozen specific forms of autophagy, but for the purpose of a higher consciousness perspective, I am going to focus on "macro autophagy," which is the main degradation pathway that breaks down damaged cells and proteins. This occurs by creating a double membrane autophagosome around the damaged cell or protein and directing it into a lysosome, where the degraded or damaged cell or protein will be destroyed. This metabolic process then converts the cellular debris and dysfunctional organelles into *energy*. It's a form of cellular alchemy.

We can think of autophagy as being determined by the nutrient status of your cells. Your body first searches for energy sources readily available in its system. If there is a steady source of food coming in, the body will always choose the path of least resistance and metabolize those sources for energy. Any excess energy not quickly gone through will be stored as fat. This also means that any damaged cells or proteins remain in our body because we cease to give the body an opportunity to repair and heal itself due to our constant eating and stored fat as energy reserves. Sometimes a fast of at least forty-eight hours is needed to push the body into a catabolic state, or self-eating state, rather than its normal metabolic state in order for repair and healing to commence.

Depending on your diet, it will take between twenty-four and seventy-two hours of fasting for autophagy to commence. You can test your pH and blood glucose levels with affordable over-the-counter dip sticks and a standard glucose meter in order to maintain healthy levels. A pH level of 7 is generally considered balanced, and a blood sugar level between 70 to 90 is considered healthy as well. During my prolonged fasts, my blood sugar would hover in the high 40s, 50s, and 60s. Your pH will also indicate when your liver is releasing large to extra-large ketones, and that is a great indicator that you are in ketosis and autophagy has commenced. Resistance training also stimulates autophagy, and it appears to me that intervals of thirty seconds of intense exercise (like running up flights of stairs or doing push-ups) with up to three minutes of rest seem to trigger all sorts of positive benefits for the growth, repair, and healing of the body. You can do these thirty-second intervals in sets of three, five, seven, and even up to ten based upon how you feel and your fitness level. I have done walking and resistance training during my prolonged fasts, and the benefits of resistance training as it pertains to autophagy is significantly greater than aerobic activity.

We have abdicated our innate ability and personal responsibility for our own health to so-called science, genetic diseases, low-frequency habits, chronic disorders, toxic thought, self-loathing, and destructive behavioral patterns. All of this disharmony can be greatly reduced, if not eliminated, through proper prolonged fasting, which triggers autophagy. Remember, your sentience has dominion over your body of energy, if it seizes it, no matter what the body's current state or hereditary tendencies are. Sentience must firmly anchor itself in its own direct and tangible presence. The immortal Self must drive the physical vehicle and its body of energy, not the egoic identity. Addictions, too, like all things, must die off when they cease to get the energy needed to exist. They cannot run their disharmonious rogue program of imperfection without your compliance, and autophagy is a powerful counterpunch to our human misprogramming.

Stem Cell

When a human embryo is initially co-created, the first cell is a type of undifferentiated stem cell, meaning it is pure potential. Nothing has been determined. All possibilities exist. The first few cells are all like this. Nothing has been determined, just more pure potentiality.

This is the physical manifestation of Source Point or Creator Consciousness energy and the limitless freedom of pure potentiality inherent in all existence—including You. These first few cells must get an electronic signal to become differentiated—to become something. This electronic symbol is desire. It is desire and then intention that directs all life in every way, and this applies to your health, repair, healing, liberation, and eventual self-mastery.

After five days of fasting, I observed, from my own higher consciousness perspective, healing from stem cell activity and reproduction within my nervous system. Prolonged fasting combined with focused intention supercharges repair and healing. Without the intake of physical food, our intention is more powerful because our body does not have to process any other information besides our powerful intention. Tangible repair and healing was taking place in my upper spine, pelvis, bladder, left leg, and foot.

My initial prolonged fast was for fourteen days. I then had one small five hundred calorie meal and undertook another seven days of fasting. Since then, I consume one meal every twenty-four to forty-eight hours as a lifestyle. I was diagnosed with type 1 diabetes, but this practice helped manage it. My A1C level, when last tested, was 5.1, which is lower than pre-diabetes. I no longer have indicators of this disease.

I logged my internal observations from a higher consciousness perspective. The following information is time-stamped in terms of what I observed:

- Weight loss begins after 36 hours of fasting.
- Fat burning starts 13 hours after fasting.
- Growth hormone is activated 13 hours after fasting.
- Detox occurs within 16–24 hours of fasting.
- Autophagy occurs at roughly 24–72 hours of fasting (depends on a person's diet).
- Self-control begins after 72 hours of fasting.
- New eating behavioral patterns are "grooved" within your body of energy after 17 days.
- Stem cells are activated/created after 120 hours of fasting.

All of these are malleable, based upon the force of will, state of consciousness, and quality of sentience. Remember, the point of all experience is to tangibly know thyself. No matter what background is playing on the green screen of our consciousness, the challenge is to experience the Self no matter what "movie" is playing in the background. Many people use food as a perpetual distraction from experiencing the Self directly. Remember, if we can observe it, it cannot be us.

We have been so thoroughly inverted due to our low frequency on Earth that we lead with our obsessive and disharmonious programming. Any inward-focused attention, which leads to Self-awareness, seems completely foreign and frightening to the egoic identity. The very thought of "I deserve to indulge in whatever I want" of this low frequency is a product of your belief-based egoic identity, not the Self. The voice in your head will literally say anything and everything to keep you from the inner recognition of your innate perfection, divinity, completeness, and love. Amazing, right?

There is a certain perfect balancing point—where yin meets yang—within the astral body (what some have called the subconscious) that reflects the image that we deeply hold of ourselves. This will be the outward physical appearance we project into the material world. In other words, a person can fast for a prolonged period of time, even make it a permanent lifestyle, but if the residual image of the self within the astral body is of being overweight or even muscular, then that is how the body of energy will be projected within the physical, regardless of the length of fast. Some people rarely eat and can be overweight or even muscular. This is an example of the incredible power of the higher consciousness. It always informs lower-frequency perceptions and therefore creates physical reality. It also illustrates that actual health and well-being go way beyond our intellectual meanderings and physical appearance.

By combining a practice of safe and supervised, prolonged fasting, along with turning off the program of illness that we are currently running, we supercharge our repair and healing like never before.

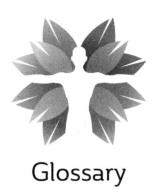

Glossary

action: The *perception* of movement. All actions are performed by an actor (the human character), but what directs action (the divine intelligence of the Self) does not move.

ascension: The moving "up" in frequencies while incarnate; the raising of the personal or collective vibration.

astral body: An aspect of the Total Self's larger energetic field or body of energy that exists within higher frequencies and outside of physical sensory perceptions. It contains the complete history of all impressions and imprints from every single stimulus upon its body of energy as well as every single creation produced, including thought, emotion, action, and behavior from every incarnation. It is the blueprint for your physical form and typically the form we project when disincarnate.

awareness: Pure, unsullied perception itself sans analysis; the eyes of the immortal Self. Embedded within pure awareness, action takes place. It is the Self's depth of unconditional love and timeless wisdom, which is sentience. Attention automatically activates the divine intelligence, or sentience, within the fabric of awareness itself.

being: Any individualized unit of consciousness, self-awareness, or sentience that was created organically through the natural attraction of like charged energies drawn together, which forms a larger, more capable and robust individual unit. Not the same as an entity, which is a manipulated creation by a higher intelligence.

being-ness: The vibratory state of an entity or being; can refer to the level of awareness of an entity or being as well.

chakra: An energy metabolizer/transformer along the human energy field. These twelve main energy interpreters (five in the front, five in the back, one atop the head, and one below the groin) draw in and translate subtle energy from outside the realm of physical perception in order to sustain and maintain the structural integrity, as well as the performance, of the human vehicle.

concept: The meanderings of limited understanding born of fragmentary sensory data; a product of the finite mind, or limited human intellect.

consciousness: The rudimentary intelligent life force that animates energy. Consciousness is expressed in infinite degrees and amounts. Consciousness has the potentiality of evolving and becoming self-aware through the accumulation and comingling of other similarly charged energies. This leads to consciousness potentially becoming self-aware, which can, in turn, lead to the development of sentient self-awareness. Sentience accrues via experiences through the use of imagination.

cosmic consciousness: An extraordinarily rare state of being and awareness that allows one access to higher frequencies, dimensional constructs, and environments within *and* outside the multiverse; cosmic consciousness affects *all* of existence in the most profound way. Buddha, Christ, Merlin, St. Germain, Plato, Babaji, and Paramahansa Yogananda are examples of cosmic consciousness.

desire: The primal life force that is utilized for the creative process itself in order for existence to understand itself. The order of creation starts with desire.

dimension: A structural component within the multiverse that measures volume like height, width, and weight. It houses the numerous frequencies within a full dimension. What we are experiencing are frequencies, not dimensions.

ego/mind/identity (EMI): The ego/mind/identity (EMI) has been commonly referred to as the ego, or ego mind, or false identity. The belief-based egoic mind is the individual's self-created totality of misperceptions, misunderstandings, and misidentifications. This includes the Self's misidentification with the perceiver and experiencer of sensory perceptions, the physical body, which binds its awareness within the confining delusion of limiting body consciousness. Every sensory perception is then seen and subsequently decoded only in relation to the false self-program running. The egoic mind is a limitation program, since all sensory perceptions are limited, and therefore so is the logic-based and linear-bound intellect. It is a product of a low-frequency environment, and its primary resultant side effect produces a stupor-like state we call thinking. *It is a limitation program that runs by thinking.*

emotion: Energy in motion based upon identification with phenomena such as thoughts, images, and experiences. The more we see the false self in it, the more we bathe the experience in emotion. This occurs in a near-instantaneous arrangement (because of the deep programming of the ego/mind/identity) of core hierarchical beliefs regarding the foundational elements of its *personal* relationship with the thought or image. The more emotional the reaction, the greater the sense of identification to the false self as it relates to the image, thought, memory, or experience.

energetic templates: The true building blocks of physical form, which exist in frequencies well outside our physical sensory perceptions. They contain the Total Self's entire past and possible pasts as well as all possible presents. There are ten templates that comprise the human form, and seven correspond to the seven main chakras. (The front and rear five main chakras correspond to a singular energetic template, as does the one crown and one root chakra.)

energy: Life substance that carries the potentiality of infinite possibility.

enlightenment: Self-realization; a varied state of being in which the Self is in communication with its Totality, or what has been referred to as the Higher Self, Godhead, or Oversoul, as well as the environment its Totality resides within. Enlightenment is different for everyone, as every Self has a unique amount, weight, and quality of sentience, as does its Totality, or Higher Self.

entity: Any individualized unit of consciousness, sentience, or sentient self-awareness that was intentionally created by others. Technically, the Total Self (what we previously referred to as the Soul) is an entity created by its Totality, or Higher Self. Humans are entities created by their Total Self. The Total Self is an entity created by its Totality, or Higher Self. Our Totality, or Higher Self, is a creation of our Source, or Creator, which makes it an entity as well. Our Source, or Creator, was created by the Absolute, or the All There Is, which makes our Source and other Sources entities as well.

exit point: A built-in potential termination event or juncture for the ending of an incarnation within the Self's life plan. The Self that incarnates as human tends to have seven potential exit points within their life plan that they can choose to avail themselves of, including prior to physical birth (as a fetus).

finite mind: The intellect. The realm of limited sensory-perceived data accessed through the five physical senses of the temporary genetic entity (body) is what creates the finite mind and its subsequent mental machinations. The extremely limited data stream provided by the physical senses is the fragmented information that creates the programs of logic and linearity, which are subprograms of the imaginary confines of space and time. The resultant fragmented conclusions that the finite mind produces are what we call facts. Facts are the imaginary fodder for the realm of so-called knowledge. Knowledge is simply the grandest of delusions. Because of these inherent limitations, the finite mind is not capable of accessing or perceiving "what is," as "what is" exists well beyond the perception of the physical senses and the logic/linear-based processing. All mental machinations are simply the meanderings of the finite mind, or thought itself.

form factor: The physical vehicle, type of body, genetic entity, or biological suit. Sentience (the Self) temporarily merges with a form factor for the purpose of incarnation within the physical universe.

freedom: The ever-present original and natural state of existence; non-identification; transcendence from misperceptions, misunderstandings, and misidentifications from the tyranny of the finite mind and its identification with the physical body; a wholly cleansed mind; non-thought. Pure awareness is the freedom inherent in limitless imagination.

free will: The "experience" of freedom as it pertains to *perceivable* choices in order to evolve oneself; the human experiment is the experiment in individualized free will as an avenue for the most expedient route for the evolution of individual and collective consciousness, or, more specifically, for the accrual of sentience; at the deepest levels, it is an illusion, as once creation is set into motion, absolute free will is no longer possible.

frequency: An assignation of energy; a specific rate or environment that energy exists within and vibrates in accordance with.

genetic entity: The physical body or vehicle; the biological suit or temporary electronic garment the Self adorns in order to protect itself and experience the lower frequencies of the physical universe. Encoded within the DNA structure is the history of every behavioral, emotional, and cultural pattern of every entity that ever physically occupied and contributed that specific genetic line of physical vehicle. The genetic entity, or what we call the "physical" body, has its own separate level of consciousness apart from the sentience and energy of the Total Self that currently occupies it. Each system, organ, and cell within the genetic entity has its own level of consciousness, and it runs based upon the programming that has been encoded within it previously.

gnosis: Direct, tangible self-knowledge. The only true knowledge is knowledge of Self—gnosis. Everything else is an opinion.

(the) Greater Reality: That which eternally exists and resides beyond our limited sensory perceptions and therefore the meanderings of the intellect.

hereditary line: The physical traits, characteristics, and tendencies within a specific genetic line of a form factor, physical vehicle, genetic entity, or biological suit.

higher intuitive functions: The expressions, attributes, abilities, or "talents" of the Self, such as clairsentience, claircognizance, clairvoyance, telepathy, etc.

hive mind: The opposite of individualized free will; collective group thinking.

identification (misidentification): The cause of all *suffering*; the misunderstanding that occurs when infinite Creator Awareness, such as the Self, misidentifies itself with *anything* that can be perceived, such as beliefs, thoughts, emotions, experiences, memories, or what has been learned. This includes the "perceiver" and "experiencer" of sensory perceptions, the genetic entity, as well as the meanderings of the intellect.

incarnate: The temporary experience that a collective life force, self-aware being, or conscious entity has within the lower frequencies of the physical universe.

Intelligent Energy (IE): Energy that vibrates at frequencies above the realm of physical perception. Higher frequential Intelligent Energy, due to its more holistic nature and environment, naturally harmonizes, repairs, and heals energy that vibrates within lower frequencies.

intention: The harnessing of energy, or qi; a fixed focal point of energy within the creative process.

judgment: The opposite of unconditional love; nonacceptance; the belief-based ego/mind/identity; the egoic false self imposing its sense of self upon the divine Self, others, and all sensory-perceived stimuli.

knowledge: Justified beliefs; a form of hypnosis; the woefully incomplete set of conclusions based upon fragmented sensory-perceived data processed by the limitations of the logical and linear-based intellect; the accumulation of information in order to become capable of performing a repetitious task that is bound by time. Knowledge belongs to the realm of temporary personhood, which is why it cannot touch that which is eternal. Knowledge is simply the grandest form of ignorance and arrogance, a delusion. A key component of the belief-based egoic mind.

(the) Law of Cause and Effect: That which is set into motion and gathers similar energies, all of which eventually returns to its source point in order for the original creator to fully understand what it has given birth to. *Only* the wisdom born of unconditional love operates above this immutable and eternal law of the universe. A being that operates at this level is a being of pure cause sans effect. A Master.

(the) Law of Karma: The deep misidentification and subsequent attachment to anything low-frequency (desire, intention, thought, emotion, action, and behavior). This attachment creates a literal electric connection that binds the higher-dimensional Self to the lower frequencies of the physical universe, thus imprisoning it until the attachment is severed. The attachment can be undone only within the realm in which it was created. The attachment to any strictly human behavior creates karma.

Light: The physical representation of spirit; a fractal of Source/God/Creator; loving, divine intelligence itself.

magick: The ability to harness and manipulate higher frequential energies that exist beyond physical sensory perceptions by utilizing pure desire and unbroken intention. This can be augmented by the use of higher intuitive functions.

Marlon and Sophia: My companion entity who is presently embodied as two Jack Russell/Chihuahua mixes and previously as my first dog, Clyde. They are both aspects of the same larger Totality/Higher Self that is always with me, in one form or multiple forms, whenever I incarnate in the physical universe.

Master: A true timeless teacher of humanity; a fully God-realized being.

meditation: The space between thoughts; the cessation of the egoic mind running its program of limitations we call thinking. When done properly, meditation annihilates the misperception that we are merely human or limited in any way. The freeing of awareness from ordinary sensory perceptions, the limiting intellect, and debilitating body consciousness.

metaphysics: Hidden from the five senses and therefore the processing of the logical and linear intellect are the inner workings, depth, function, and interplay of sentience and energy; a more holistic and accurate understanding of existence itself.

multi-frequential: Energy and/or sentience that simultaneously exists within multiple frequencies concurrently and in parallel.

(the) Old Religion: The ancient practices and understandings of the nature of the Greater Reality and how to harness it for transmutation and transcendence (what has been referred to as alchemy).

(the) Original You: The pure sentience and energy unsullied by low frequency experience; perfection, divinity, and freedom itself; the harmonized and perfectly balanced individualized unit of God/Source/Creator prior to becoming astray; the non-disharmonious state of the Self, which has been made disharmonious through incarnating in order to participate within the evolutionary cycle.

phenomena/phenomenon: Any sense perception, which includes the incarnation itself, and everything the incarnation perceives, including but not limited to belief, thought, emotions, actions, behaviors, and the body itself.

(the) Real You: The Self.

reality: The self-directed relationship an individual creates in regard to all sensory stimuli; individualized, group, or collective experience seen from a similar state of understanding.

Reiki: A very ancient healing modality originally created by an Ascended Master in which the practitioner, through the harnessing of their intention, uses their energetic and physical body as a conduit of higher-frequency energy for healing aided by the utilization of specific symbols.

Self: Sentience; the amount, level, or weight of our love and wisdom.

self-inquiry: The direct introspection into the nature of the Self.

Self-mastery: The Self, while projected from its Totality, existing in a state of knowing *itself* at the very depths and origination of its existence during its incarnation; the ability to transcend the self-imposed limitations of the egoic mind, body consciousness, and localized frequential environment, as well as the ability to command energies within and outside the Total Self at will. This exalted state is always in direct proportion and relation to the level or amount of sentience that is the Self. Authentic Self-mastery is an extraordinarily rare occurrence and is the domain of very specific incarnations of Masters.

sensory perceptions: That which is perceived via the five physical senses, which can include the phenomena perceived through higher intuitive functions.

sentience: What we really are; the Self; the amount, level, or weight of timeless wisdom and unconditional love expressed as an individualized unit or collective; divine, loving intelligence not bound by space or time.

Soul: See *Total Self.* The individualized unit comprised of both sentience and its complement of energy; sentience and energy are always in a direct one-to-one ratio to each other.

Source: Our Creator, or God. We exist *within* Source's creation called the multiverse, which is *within* Source itself. Everything within our entire multiverse is a creation, whether direct or indirect, of our Source, with the tiniest of exceptions we call the Ascended Masters.

spiritual materialism: Misperceptions, misunderstandings, and misidentifications as they relate to spirituality; The egoic mind's hallucinatory desire to become, achieve, and acquire as it relates to spirituality or esoteric information; its desire to find, experience, and potentially possess so-called higher esoteric knowledge, which can include bodily sensations; its pursuit of both the tangible and the intangible as it relates to spiritual belief systems.

suffering: The self-created experience of disharmony brought on by misperceptions, misunderstandings, and misidentifications; humanity's preferred method for the evolution of its consciousness. The experience of suffering was created in order for the Self to fully understand and therefore appreciate what it eternally is: love.

thought: The movement of the past; the movement of memory, experience, and so-called knowledge. All thought is the past, including the so-called future, as the past must be recalled in order to conceptualize a future. Thinking is faltering itself and is simply a by-product of experiencing a low-frequency environment—the opposite of knowing.

Total Self: Sentience—what we really are—given a complement or body of energy to create with; our individualized sentience and its complement of energy projected from our Totality. What we totally are even while incarnate—not the person within the human experience, but what originally gives birth to any temporary experiences of personhood, including personhood itself. Commonly referred to as the Soul.

Totality/Higher Self: The much larger being that we are a tiny projection of. Our Totality is everything we have been, are, and will be. The Total Self (Soul) is but a mere drop of its Totality. Our

Totality exists well beyond the constructs of time and space, and based upon its degree, amount, or weight of sentience, determines which of the twelve dimensions it resides in within the multiverse. Commonly referred to as the Higher Self, Godhead, or Oversoul.

transcendence: The moving into a more holistic state of awareness; a rise in frequential beingness beyond a limited understanding of that which is currently experienced.

transmutation: The enhancement, or augmentation, from that which is into that which can be; the foundation of alchemy.

(the) True Self: See the *Self.*

wisdom: The direct, experiential knowingness that occurs only though observation; the divine intelligence of the Self; the timeless knowingness that is part of the very fabric of the immortal Self; the eternally applicable level of gnosis woven within the fabric of awareness itself.

To Write to the Author

If you wish to contact the author or would like more information about this book, please write to the author in care of Llewellyn Worldwide Ltd. and we will forward your request. Both the author and the publisher appreciate hearing from you and learning of your enjoyment of this book and how it has helped you. Llewellyn Worldwide Ltd. cannot guarantee that every letter written to the author can be answered, but all will be forwarded. Please write to:

RJ Spina
℅ Llewellyn Worldwide
2143 Wooddale Drive
Woodbury, MN 55125-2989
Please enclose a self-addressed stamped envelope for reply,
or $1.00 to cover costs. If outside the U.S.A., enclose
an international postal reply coupon.

Many of Llewellyn's authors have websites with additional information and resources. For more information, please visit our website at http://www.llewellyn.com.